PROFESSIONAL CURIOSITY IN SAFEGUARDING ADULTS

PROFESSIONAL CURIOSITY IN SAFEGUARDING ADULTS

Ann Anka, Helen Thacker, Bridget Penhale, Walter Lloyd-Smith and Becky Booth

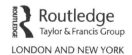

LONDON AND NEW YORK

Cover design by Out of House

First published 2025
by Routledge
4 Park Square, Milton Park, Abingdon, Oxon OX14 4RN

and by Routledge
605 Third Avenue, New York, NY 10158

Routledge is an imprint of the Taylor & Francis Group, an informa business

© 2025 Ann Anka, Becky Booth, Walter Lloyd-Smith, Bridget Penhale and Helen Thacker

The right of Ann Anka, Becky Booth, Walter Lloyd-Smith, Bridget Penhale and Helen Thacker to be identified as authors of this work has been asserted in accordance with sections 77 and 78 of the Copyright, Designs and Patents Act 1988.

All rights reserved. No part of this book may be reprinted or reproduced or utilised in any form or by any electronic, mechanical, or other means, now known or hereafter invented, including photocopying and recording, or in any information storage or retrieval system, without permission in writing from the publishers.

Trademark notice: Product or corporate names may be trademarks or registered trademarks, and are used only for identification and explanation without intent to infringe.

British Library Cataloguing in Publication Data
A CIP record for this book is available from the British Library

ISBN: 9781041056607 (hbk)
ISBN: 9781916925205 (pbk)
ISBN: 9781041056591 (ebk)

DOI: 10.4324/9781041056591

Text design by Greensplash
Typeset in ITC Franklin Gothic Book
by Newgen Publishing UK

Contents

	Acknowledgements	*vi*
	About the authors	*vii*
	Foreword	*x*
	Introduction: Professional curiosity and safeguarding adult practice	1
1	What is professional curiosity?	5
2	Barriers to professional curiosity in safeguarding adults	23
3	Enablers of professional curiosity in safeguarding adult practice	44
4	Application of professional curiosity to practice	65
5	The legal and policy context of partnership work in safeguarding adults	84
6	Putting partnership work into practice	104
7	Conclusion	122
	References	*141*
	Index	*159*

Acknowledgements

We would like to thank friends, families, colleagues and mentors for their support and encouragement. A special thanks goes to Leanne Rhodes (University of East Anglia) for her timeless support and to all at Critical Publishing, especially Di Page, Julia Morris, Lily Harrison and Annie Rose, for their support for, and advice about, the book.

About the authors

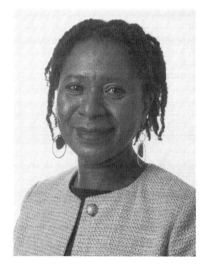

Ann Anka

Ann Anka is an Associate Professor in Social Work at the University of East Anglia (UEA). Her specialist area of practice is social work with adults. She has taught on safeguarding adults and adult social care law at undergraduate, postgraduate and Continuing Professional Development (CPD) levels in England. She has also developed and led two CPD modules for qualified social workers: one centres on safeguarding adults and the other on dementia care. Her research interests are on service user and carer involvement in social work and on safeguarding adults, particularly adults with hoarding difficulties. Ann has a professional qualification in social work and social policy. She worked as a social worker at the London Borough Havering before entering academia. She is a trustee at Abbeyfield Norwich, a residential care home for older people.

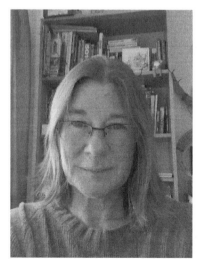

Becky Booth

Becky Booth is a deputy manager with Safeguarding Adults Boards at Norfolk. She is a registered social worker. Becky has worked in adult social care since 1994. She worked as a Safeguarding Adults practice consultant prior to taking up her current position. She has over ten years' experience in supporting social care staff, partner agency colleagues and providers in section 42 *Care Act 2014* enquiries and associated safeguarding work across all specialisations.

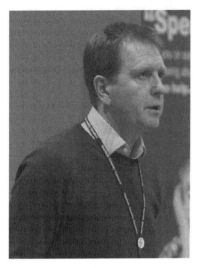

Walter Lloyd-Smith

Walter Lloyd-Smith has a professional qualification in occupational therapy. He has been a manager and business lead for Norfolk Safeguarding Adults Board since 2015. He previously worked for five years as the Safeguarding Adults Lead for a community health provider. He developed this role from scratch, supporting the board and staff across the organisation, from frontline to the senior management team, to meet their obligations to safeguard adults at risk of abuse and harm. Walter worked in a range of services including physical health, mental health in-patients and forensic services before moving to work in a physical disability team with social services. He previously worked as a research assistant for the Cambridgeshire Elders Occupational Therapy Trial, a DoH-funded, community-based, randomised control trial hosted by UEA between 1999 and 2002.

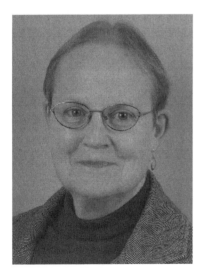

Bridget Penhale

Bridget Penhale is an Emeritus Professor in health sciences at UEA. She has an extensive research and practice knowledge and understanding of safeguarding adults. She has also published extensively on partnership work and safeguarding adults. She has written blogs on cases heard at the Open Justice Court of Protection. Among her research interests are elder abuse, including institutional forms of abuse; adult safeguarding (also known as adult protection or adult abuse); intimate partner violence/domestic violence; attachment and intergenerational relationships in later life; the mental health of older people; loss, grief and bereavement in later life; adult social care and community care; ethics and social care; and health-related social work. With a first degree in psychology, Bridget has a professional qualification in social work and clinical experience in a range of settings, including health-related organisations. Following extensive experience as a social worker and (frontline) manager, the latter part of her career was spent in academic settings, with a specialist focus in gerontology.

Helen Thacker

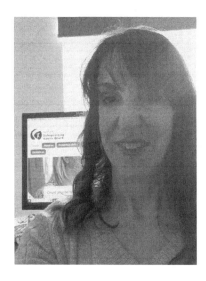

Helen Thacker is Head of Service for Safeguarding Adults at Norfolk County Council and is a registered social worker. She is a member of the county's Safeguarding Adults Board and its Safeguarding Adults Review Group. She has a particular interest in systems thinking and the application of learning from neuroscience in relation to safeguarding and curiosity. She contributes to the teaching of medical students at the University of East Anglia's School of Medicine and has published in several peer-reviewed journals.

Foreword

We are so lucky that our work and our professional values encourage and support us to be curious as curiosity drives our learning, and learning stimulates our curiosity. I would argue that professional curiosity is essential for everyone working in social care and health, as well as those working in the many organisations and sectors concerned with safeguarding adults.

We would not be in these roles if we did not care about the people we work with and for, and want to know about their lives. This is important to understand how best to support people so they can keep themselves safe and be in control of their own lives. I know from years of work promoting the Making Safeguarding Personal approach, that resolution and recovery from abuse and neglect requires working in a personalised way, which involves finding out what someone wants to happen in their lives to be safe. This is what will make a protection plan effective and achieve both safety and well-being for the person involved. In order to do this, professional curiosity is essential. We should also be fiercely committed to relating to the people we work with in the same way we would want our friends and family members to be treated by professionals: being curious with sensitivity and respect, and mindful of our duties of care.

This book is unique in explaining how and why professional curiosity is essential to what we do in safeguarding adults, and how and why we do it. It shows how professional curiosity can be nurtured and encouraged, as well as blocked and stifled. It explores what we have learned from a raft of evidence, including Safeguarding Adult Reviews, when professional curiosity was lacking, with such human cost. In a changing environment with multiple challenges, to understand how professional curiosity operates – including what helps and hinders – means we can consider how we can support and develop professional curiosity in ourselves and others.

Although primarily aimed at students, this book is essential reading for those of us who are concerned about how to develop and improve the ways in which we deliver our safeguarding responsibilities. We can all learn from the depth and breadth of knowledge and insight contained in these pages. It is a practical endeavour, prompting the reader to reflect on their own assumptions and behaviours. It uses case studies from a wide range of situations, reflections from people with lived experience, to enhance understanding of how professional curiosity works, what it means for each of us personally and what impact it has when applied properly and effectively.

The team who has written this book has modelled the collaborative and partnership approach that is essential in all safeguarding adults' work. Their knowledge and insights are well articulated and accessible. Whoever we are, whatever our experience of safeguarding adults, we can always learn more.

Dr Adi Cooper OBE
Independent safeguarding Consultant
Independent Consultant – safeguarding adults
and adult social care
March 2025

Introduction: Professional curiosity and safeguarding adult practice

Professional curiosity is an essential element in professional practice across the range of professions such as social work, nursing and midwifery, occupational therapy, police and probation services. Professional curiosity is viewed as a model of practice, an approach and a behavioural attribute. It comprises knowledge, skills and values, as well as the ability to listen, ask questions and not take things at face value. It involves asking further questions for clarity, perspective talking and perspective listening (we explore these concepts in more depth in Chapter 6; for further reading, see Calvard et al, 2023). In addition, professional curiosity involves skills and the ability to assess, identify and manage risks in a co-productive way. It also includes the ability to build relationships of trust and work with others, including those who may be hard to like. Moreover, it involves the use of self and intuition; the ability to use evidence to support one's initial thoughts; the ability to reflect, use critical thinking and analyse; the ability to make judgements and decisions, while being culturally aware; and the use of compassion and kindness to respectfully challenge when necessary.

Professional curiosity is central to safeguarding adult practice. Safeguarding adults is enshrined in law and centres on supporting the rights of people to live safely, free from abuse, harm and neglect. In the United Kingdom, policy tells us that safeguarding adults is 'everyone's responsibility'. Practitioners and organisations are required to work together to safeguard those at risk or who have experienced harm, abuse and neglect. Importantly, Safeguarding Adult Reviews (SARs), Children Safeguarding Practice Reviews (CSPRs) and analysis of Domestic Abuse Related Death Reviews (DARDRs) into the deaths of adults and children that have resulted from violence, abuse, neglect and harm often cite a lack of professional curiosity as key to failing to protect those owed the duty of care and protection from abuse, neglect and harm.

Why write this book?

Policy and law require that those engaged in safeguarding work, including those training to work in the field of safeguarding adult practice, employ professional curiosity. This book seeks to raise awareness about the importance of professional curiosity in safeguarding adult practice. Professional, Statutory and Regulatory Bodies (PSRBs) require that those training or studying to work in safeguarding adult practice develop, maintain and use professional curiosity. Yet no books currently exist to guide those in training and or studying on PSRB courses on what the concept of professional curiosity entails, and the practice skills required to engage in professional curiosity practice. The book is therefore timely. At the time of writing, in the spring of 2024, our research found that there is no book in social work with adults, nursing and midwifery, occupational therapy and other allied health and social care professions with a focus on professional curiosity. This also includes the police, professionals from the criminal justice system, except for probation services, which has a practitioner's guide that focuses specifically on professional curiosity in safeguarding adult practice.

The Covid-19 pandemic has significantly changed and impacted the systems and structures that support us – including different ways of working. These changes have had a significant impact on effective engagement in professional curiosity practice, both negatively and positively. It is now harder to get appointments with professionals, people are having to wait longer for appointments, and they are often seen only when they have reached a crisis point. Due to continuing austerity measures across the United Kingdom, we also have fewer resources to support an ageing population. Other changes include remote working, which is now the norm. Most initial screening assessments are now carried out remotely by telephone or via digital platforms such as Zoom or Microsoft (MS) Teams. Most professional meetings also take place remotely via such digital platforms. While many of these changes to ways of working via digital platforms are good, back-to-back Zoom or MS Teams meetings without breaks can affect our cognitive abilities to ask curious questions due to tiredness. On a more positive note, remote work offers opportunities for different professionals to come together to share knowledge and resources, far more quickly than in pre-pandemic times. The Open Justice Court of Protection has demonstrated the capacity to harness digital technology not only in the court system but also for reaching a wider audience. Aside from the new ways of working, new legislation has been introduced, such as reforms of mental health law, while others have been paused. These may all have a retrospective effect on safeguarding adults work. There is therefore a need to know about these changes in order to protect the rights of those at risk or experiencing abuse, harm and neglect.

This book seeks to raise awareness about the importance of professional curiosity in safeguarding adult practice. It is an introductory book, it engages the reader in critical reflection on what professional curiosity is, why professional curiosity is important in safeguarding adults and what the practice skills are, together with the attributes, values and legal literacy required for professional curiosity practice, what has changed and what has not since the pandemic. The aim is to share our thoughts and perspectives on what professional curiosity is by drawing from our practice experiences and from the broad literature, research – including safeguarding adults reviews (SARs) – law and policy. We also invite you, the reader, to share your thoughts and perspectives about your engagement in professional curiosity practice with others – colleagues, peers (including those at the centre of safeguarding concerns), their families and carers – as you read this book. We want everyone to know about the importance of using professional curiosity in everyday (working) lives, and the barriers and facilitators – including the resources needed to do so. We want participation in professional curiosity to be a daily routine in our engagement with others to help us to work together to save lives and enhance well-being.

Who is the book written for?

This book is intended primarily for undergraduate and postgraduate students, including apprentices studying qualifying courses. This includes, for example, those studying social work, newly qualified social workers, allied health and social care professions, students in nursing and midwifery and occupational therapy, those working in the criminal justice system, police and probation and all involved in safeguarding adult work. In addition, experienced and qualified practitioners who work in safeguarding adult practice would find the book useful, as would practice educators (those supervising students on placements or field education). The book also appeals to practitioners with an interest in safeguarding adults more generally, particularly those working in adult social care. Academic researchers and practitioner-researchers engaged in safeguarding adults, particularly on professional curiosity, would also find it useful.

Key features of the book

The book is written in plain English, from both academic and practice perspectives. All the chapters are interactive and include case study activities drawn from SARs and practice, together with reflective questions. In addition, key summary/action points and suggested further readings are included to enable you to consider the key messages discussed in the chapters and what to take forward. You are invited throughout the book, as an active participant, to test your knowledge and understanding, and to engage in critical reflections on using professional curiosity in safeguarding adult work. The book also introduces you to other books within the series where you can learn about specific topics such as policy, law and the skills required for practice in depth. We encourage you, as an active participant, to reflect on the knowledge gained, to seek out further learning and to engage in learning with others – including learning with and from people who use services, those with eligible needs and those without – and to apply the knowledge gained to your practice.

Structure of the book

The book has seven main chapters in addition to this introductory chapter. It covers the concept of curiosity and professional curiosity, core skills and attributes needed for professional curiosity practice and the legal and policy context of safeguarding adults, including partnership work.

Chapter 1 explores the concept of curiosity, what is meant by professional curiosity, why it is important in safeguarding adult practice and implications for failing to engage in professional curiosity practice. The chapter includes core skills and attributes required for professional curiosity practice in safeguarding those owed a duty of care and protection from abuse, neglect and harm.

Chapter 2 considers barriers to effective professional curiosity in safeguarding adults, drawing from lessons to be learnt from practice, children safeguarding practice reviews and safeguarding adult reviews. The chapter hones in on practitioner responsibilities, particularly the role of managers and agencies with responsibilities for safeguarding adults.

Chapter 3 focuses on enablers of professional curiosity practice in safeguarding adults by exploring individual and organisational factors that interact to produce conditions favourable to a curious, inquiring approach. These are examined through the lens of neuroscience as well as practice frameworks.

Chapter 4 focuses on the skills, attributes and values required for engaging in professional curiosity practice in work undertaken with those owed a duty of care and protection from abuse, neglect and harm and their families and carers, including service user and carer participation.

Chapter 5 centres on the legal and policy context of partnership work in safeguarding adults and professional curiosity practice. The chapter focuses on why partnership work is important in safeguarding adults. This is examined from the legal requirements to work with other professionals as well as the requirement to involve people who use services. The chapter explores the legal and policy framework in England. Comparisons are made between the four countries of the United Kingdom and other international jurisdictions.

Chapter 6 looks at the skills, attributes and values required for partnership work with those owed a duty of care and protection from abuse, neglect and harm, and their families and carers and other professionals. The chapter considers new ways of working in a post-pandemic world and how to harness the opportunities of using digital technology to connect with others as well as support those owed a duty of care, including practice implications.

Chapter 7 includes useful guidance on risk identification and assessments, and provides practice tools to undertake risk assessments. It pulls together the central arguments of the book, drawing attention to the importance of using professional curiosity in safeguarding adults work and the likely consequences of failing to do so.

1 What is professional curiosity?

> **CHAPTER OBJECTIVES**
>
> **By the end of this chapter, you should be able to:**
>
> - understand what is meant by curiosity;
> - understand what professional curiosity is;
> - ascertain the importance of professional curiosity in safeguarding adult practice;
> - identify the core skills and attributes required for professional curiosity practice in safeguarding adult work.

Introduction

This chapter explores the concepts of curiosity and professional curiosity. It looks at why they are important in safeguarding adult practice, and the skills and attributes required to engage in professional curiosity in safeguarding adults who are at risk of, or are experiencing, abuse, harm and neglect. The chapter also considers organisations' responsibilities for supporting practitioners to engage in professional curiosity. We use the term 'practitioners' throughout the chapter to encapsulate the different professionals, staff, trainees, students and apprentices who have the responsibility in the course of their work to safeguard and protect adults from abuse, harm and neglect, including researchers engaged in safeguarding work. The chapter begins by explaining the concept of curiosity; this is followed by the concept of professional curiosity and why professional curiosity is important in safeguarding adult work.

Definitional considerations: what is curiosity?

The concept of curiosity is described as an information-seeking behaviour, a quest for knowledge and an innate desire to know more. Curiosity is linked to the drive or motivation to learn, to know and understand, the desire and excitement to explore new things through our interactions with others, by asking questions to gain deeper understanding about what is going on. Curiosity has also been linked to the ability to cope with and manage ambiguity and uncertainty. This relates to the uneasiness that comes with not knowing something and the intrinsic drive to seek, know, understand and find resolutions. The concept of curiosity has been defined by Kashdan et al (2018, p 130) as *'the recognition, pursuit, and desire to explore novel, uncertain, complex, and ambiguous events'*. The authors go on to suggest that when perceptual curiosity arises, *'there is the feeling of interest in a situation where a potential exists for learning. There is a desire to seek out novel experiences – to see what happens, to find out how one will react, or discover how others react'* (Kashdan et al, 2018, p 130). Curiosity has also been described as a *'human need to make ordered sense of the world'* (Kedge and Appleby, 2009, p 636), *'an impulse towards better cognition'* (Kidd and Hayden, 2015, p 450) and as personal traits or personal characteristics (Kashdan et al, 2018). Curiosity is viewed as an important motivator for learning (Berlyne, 1954; Litman and Spielberger, 2003; Loewenstein, 1994). Within the health and human sciences, it is a useful motivator for helping us understand what is going on in people's lives. Roman (2011, p 655) notes that *'curiosity allows us to dig deeper to find answers and, in the process, to listen more attentively to the fears and concerns of our patients* [service users]'. A number of attributes linked to being curious include the ability to recognise or a desire to pursue and explore unfamiliar or unclear complex events (Kashdan et al, 2018; Whitecross and Smithson, 2023). Curiosity also involves the ability and desire to question, apply critical thinking and critical evaluation skills, and reflection. Yager and Kay (2020, p 1) describe curiosity as *'a basic motivation to sense, experience, explore, and understand something which is unfamiliar, regardless of whether a tangible extrinsic reward might be attached'*. The concept of curiosity has also been linked to fear and the potential risk to which one may be exposed (Loewenstein, 1994). You might have heard of the English proverb *'curiosity kills the cat'*. Loewenstein (1994) notes that while some people may be comfortable with the uncertainties and ambiguities of not knowing about what is going on and seek to find answers, others may choose not to do so due to fear of the unknown.

As you might have gathered from these different conceptualisations, how individuals demonstrate curiosity has been the subject of many studies (eg Berlyne, 1954; Kashdan et al, 2018; Litman and Spielberger, 2003; Loewenstein, 1994). These studies have focused on the relationships between what motivates us to learn, our emotional response to learning and how these factors affect our interactions with others, the world around us and the decisions we make. Earlier conceptualisations of curiosity centred on the notion of epistemic curiosity, which refers to the desire for knowledge. Epistemic curiosity is based on two forms of curiosity: one resulting from the pleasure or the excitement that we experience when we want to learn new things; and one that develops from a desire to learn due to the frustration of not knowing in order to address an information gap (Berlyne, 1954; Loewenstein, 1994). Built on these earlier conceptualisations, the literature identifies different dimensions of curiosity, which are usually constructed round either two or five dimensions of curiosity. Researchers have developed different scales to establish how people demonstrate curiosity. The two most-discussed dimensions of curiosity are interest-type curiosity (also referred to as dispositional interest-curiosity, or curiosity as a feeling of interest) and deprivation-type curiosity (also known as curiosity-as-deprivation) (Berlyne, 1954; Litman, 2008; Litman and Jimerson, 2004). Interest-type curiosity has been described as the excitement or joy we experience when we *feel interest* in learning new information or new things. Here, we want to learn or have a desire to learn for fun, for its own sake or to gain pleasure. In contrast, deprivation-type curiosity has been described as the sense and feelings that we experience when faced with not having the information we need. This is the sense of feeling we go through when we desperately need information to put pieces together but do not have that information. Litman (2008, p 1587) describes this feeling as *'being bothered by having insufficient information'* or as what *'really gets on my nerves when I know that I am close to solving a puzzle, but still cannot figure it out'*. Litman's (2008) research found that what motivates us to learn in deprivation-type curiosity focuses on finding solutions to address specific problems. Here we seek to lower anxiety or our frustrations by finding solutions to what we do not know. We want to know not because we are interested in acquiring new knowledge; rather our curiosity comes from a desire to know in order to close an information gap. A key drawback of deprivation-type curiosity is that it includes high levels of negative emotions such as anxiety and anger. Zedelius et al's (2022, p 15) research found that those with deprivation-type curiosity had *'a promiscuous desire for information, but also a lack of humility, or openness to revising their beliefs in light of new evidence'*. Studies examining the benefits and drawbacks of the two curiosity types suggest those with deprivation-type curiosity do well in performance-orientated tasks whereas those with interest-type curiosity do well in mastery-oriented learning tasks (Ryakhovskaya et al, 2022; Whitecross and Smithson, 2023a). Building on these earlier studies, Kashdan et al's (2018) research with a sample of 3000 people identified five dimensions of curiosity and four types of curious people.

Five dimensions of curiosity

Table 1.1 presents a summary of the five dimensions of curiosity and how the dimensions manifest.

Table 1.1 A summary of the five dimensions of curiosity developed by Kashdan et al's (2018) research

The five dimensions of curiosity	Characterisation of the dimensions
Joyous exploration	This is associated with the joy and excitement we experience when we want to learn something new for its own sake and for the pleasure of learning.

The five dimensions of curiosity	Characterisation of the dimensions
Deprivation sensitivity	This is characterised by the anxiety and frustration that we go through when we do not know something, want to know it and spend time learning about what we do not know.
Stress tolerance	This is characterised by how one copes or deals with anxiety, doubts, uncertainty, ambiguity or fear when faced with learning new things, or something that challenges us.
Thrill seeking	This is characterised by risk taken just for the pleasurable experience of taking risk or not being afraid to take risk. Here, what confronts us is what gives us the desire to experience and face that risk full on. A key drawback is that if this not channelled into meaningful activities, it could lead to reckless behaviour.
Social curiosity (overt and covert social curiosity)	Relates to the desire to learn what others are thinking and doing by talking, listening and observing their behaviour. Two types of social curiosity are identified: • *Overt social curiosity:* relates to wanting to learn what others are thinking and feeling to understand how they behave. Here, social information is gathered by directly talking to people. • *Covert social curiosity:* relates to gathering information about others from friends/families/neighbours or reading about them.

Four types of curious people

Table 1.2 provides a summary of the four types of curious people identified in Kashdan et al's (2018) research, including the development of their scorings on a five dimensions of curiosity scale. They provide fascinating insights into what motivates us to learn and our emotional responses including drawbacks.

Table 1.2 A summary of the four types of curious people identified in Kashdan et al's (2018) research

Four types of curious people	Characteristics – scoring: What do we know about them?
The fascinator	Fascinators were found to be highly curious; they do not get stressed easily. They are described as possessing the psychological strength to explore, discover and have sustained interests, and are persistent in seeking or acquiring new knowledge. They scored highest on Joyous Exploration, Stress Tolerance, and Thrill Seeking and lowest on Deprivation Sensitivity.

Four types of curious people	Characteristics – scoring: What do we know about them?
Problem-solver	Problem-solvers were found to be highly interested in solving problems. They like to uncover something specific to address a knowledge or information gap. They value independence. They scored highest on Deprivation Sensitivity, high on Joyous Exploration, and lowest on Social Curiosity.
Empathisers	Described themselves as anxious and introverted. They often feel stressed but tended to give the impression that their lives were in control. Empathisers like to observe what is going on around them more so than participate. They have high levels of Social Curiosity and low levels of Thrill Seeking and Stress Tolerance.
Avoiders	The avoiders were found to be the least curious. They tend to steer clear of difficult and challenging situations as well as avoiding confrontation where possible. Avoiders scored low on all five dimensions, particularly on Stress Tolerance; they scored high on Deprivation Sensitivity.

REFLECTIVE QUESTIONS

- What motivates you to learn?
- What are the strengths and drawbacks of what motivates you to learn?
- Make a list of what you would do to address the drawbacks identified.
- Make a list of what you would do to build on the strengths identified.
- Write a brief reflective summary about your understanding of the concept of curiosity.
- What would you take forward from learning about the concept of curiosity?

APPLYING CONCEPTS TO PRACTICE

Kashdan et al (2018) note that engagement in curiosity helps us to expand our knowledge, build competencies, strengthen our relationships with others and increase innovation and creativity. The authors point out that a key function of curiosity is to 'seek out, explore, and immerse oneself in situations with potential for new information and/or experiences' (Kashdan et al, 2018, p 130). Drawing from this statement, consider the following case study and answer the questions.

→

> **Case study**
>
> Antonio, an 80 year-old Italian man, is referred to a community hub team for support. The referral reveals that Antonio lives with his partner Kay in an owner-occupied bungalow. He has a son who lives about 50 miles away. Antonio was diagnosed with Alzheimer's disease in 2020. He was discharged from hospital recently following a significant decline in his health. You have received a distressing phone call from Kay that Antonio has locked himself in the bathroom and is refusing to come out.

TASK

- Make a note of how you would work with Antonio and Kay in this case study.
- Decide, from the four types of curious people described by Kashdan et al (2018), what type of curious person you are.
- What have you learnt about yourself?
- What are you good at and what do you need to work more on based on what you have learnt about yourself by participating in this activity?

Why is curiosity important in safeguarding work?

The literature tells us that curiosity is context specific. Curiosity is recognised as a desirable trait in safeguarding adult practice and in professions such as social work, nursing, education, midwifery, dentistry, medical doctors, psychiatric, housing, occupational therapy, policing and probation work (BASW, 2018; Dyche and Epstein, 2011; Guthrie, 2020; HM Inspectorate of Probation, 2022; Yager and Kay, 2020). The concept of curiosity is very important for understanding what influences the actions and decisions that practitioners make when engaging in safeguarding adult practice and how our actions and decisions affect those at risk of abuse, harm and neglect. We hope that by participating in the above activities, you have been able to identify your areas of strength and areas that you need to develop further in order to use curiosity when working with others. In the next section, we explore professional curiosity.

What is professional curiosity?

The concept of professional curiosity was first alluded to in an enquiry into the death of Victoria Climbie by Lord Laming in 2003 and by the Munro Review (2010) in the United Kingdom. It is built on the premise that practitioners do not hold all information, so need to seek out what they do not know from others to understand what is going on with the person at risk of, or experiencing, abuse, harm and/or neglect. This information could be sought from individuals' families and carers as well as from other practitioners who may hold the information needed to protect the rights of those at risk of abuse to live in safety and free from abuse and harm (DHSC, 2024). The concept of professional curiosity is central to safeguarding work. Safeguarding adult practice consists of using different strategies and approaches, including duties and powers, core skills and values, to inform assessments of risk and implementations of various interventions that are aimed at protecting the rights of people to live safely free from abuse and neglect. Professional curiosity is one of the key approaches and strategies used.

Similar to the concept of curiosity, there is no single agreed definition of what professional curiosity is. Numerous definitions are offered in the literature, including in some practice guidances, on what professional curiosity is; this makes it difficult to fully define. Further, most practice literature, including enquiry reports, attributes professional curiosity to skills, traits, attributes and behaviours. Many local authorities in the United Kingdom have also offered different definitions, which draw on core skills and values required for engaging in safeguarding work in both adults and children and in family practice. These include, for example, the capacity needed to seek and clarify information when working with others to gain a deeper understanding of what is going on. For example, Thacker et al (2019, p 253) define professional curiosity as '*the capacity and communication skill to explore and understand what is happening* [in an individual's life or] *within a family rather than making assumptions or accepting things at face value in social work practice*'. In relation to young people, Williams and Chisholm (2018, p 203) note that professionally curious practice involves '*asking questions that give and solicit information without being intrusive or making the young person feel threatened. These should be open-ended and allow for additional probing.*' Through their research, Phillips et al (2022) sought the views of 445 probation workers in England and Wales about what professional curiosity meant to them and reported that most practitioners who took part associated the concept with managing risk. The concept was also viewed as useful for the development of therapeutic alliance and knowledge building (Phillips et al, 2022). Professionally curious practice is also perceived as useful in allowing practitioners to critically analyse and appraise information received in safeguarding work to identify inconsistencies or gaps, thus enabling them to seek further information where required in order to appropriate support, thereby ensuring that the person needing protection is safe. Engagement in professional curiosity in safeguarding work therefore centres on using effective communication skills and values such as empathy and respect to seek further information about what we do not know to safeguard people from abuse, neglect and harm.

Uncertainty and ambiguities exist in safeguarding adult work, and people's lives depend on our effective engagement as practitioners with capabilities and competence that at times will save lives. Participating in professional curiosity practice involves the ability to confront uncertainty as well as over-confidence. This involves the capabilities to draw from multiple perspectives to make sense of what is going in the people's lives. Burton and Revell (2018, p 1512) note that '*curiosity is characterised by growth, exploration and development*'. Being self-aware as well as having a growth mindset is crucially important in professional curiosity practice. Lord Laming (2003) encourages us to use 'respectful curiosity'. Engagement in respectful curiosity is demonstrated through genuine interest in individual stories, focusing on what is said as well as what is not said. Bansal (2016, p 43) suggests that '*respectful curiosity not only helps us to understand each unique individual patient* [service user], *it also helps us to connect with them and build the therapeutic relationship, thereby facilitating empathy'*. Bansal (2016) notes that we show interest by taking time to listen, ask questions and show empathy; we show respect by wanting to know about the individual to understand their life histories, strengths, capabilities, challenges and how they would like to be supported. Whitlock and Purington (2013) add that we show interest in participating in respectful curiosity by asking questions, in order to understand while ensuring our curiosity is satisfied in an empathic manner.

As you might have gathered from the discussions so far, the focus of what professional curiosity is has centred on the perspectives from the practice literature and research. In what follows, we explore what is meant by professional curiosity from the perspectives of people with lived experience (PWLE). We use the term 'people with lived experience' throughout the chapter/book to capture the different terminologies used to address or describe those at who receive services (eg patients, clients, service users, carers, expert by experiences, people involvement, patient involvement).

What does professional curiosity mean to people with lived experience?

The perspective of people with lived experience in safeguarding adult work is central to participation in professional curiosity practice. Ken Mason, a PWLE, provides a summary of what professional curiosity means to him. Ken is an adoptive parent. He contributes to the involvement of PWLE in social work education at an English higher education institution. Ken's summary below provides some insights into what professional curiosity means, including some of the core skills and attributes expected by PWLE.

APPLYING CONCEPTS TO PRACTICE

Case study: what is professional curiosity from the perspectives of PWLE?

For me, professional curiosity is a way of using smart thinking to unpick what is really going on in complex family dynamics. When used correctly, it can help a practitioner gain a more accurate overview of a situation when time is at a premium, thus assisting in safer outcomes for vulnerable or at-risk people.

There are many aspects to the effective use of professional curiosity, but key is an open and non-confrontational attitude towards asking probing, wondering questions. I will give an example here from my own experience of where I feel an opportunity to use professional curiosity was missed.

On an initial visit to my son and his partner preceding Child in Need proceedings, my son's partner told the social worker that she did not want to bring her daughter up the way she had been brought up. A few gently probing questions here could have established some of the complex, wider family dynamics that had fed into the issues my son and his partner faced in parenting their daughter safely. The social worker could have explored why the couple had asked me to be present at the meeting but not the maternal grandmother. It would then have been straightforward for the worker to question me to establish that I was a protective factor rather than part of the problem.

Just that one conversation using professional curiosity could have contributed to a safer eventual outcome. Unfortunately, the case needed to be stepped up to Child Protection, a process that lasted for over a year, during which time my son was not allowed to live in the family home and was only allowed to see his daughter under my supervision. I had always been clear in meetings how much my son's behaviour contributed to the volatile situation and that I was not assigning sole blame for the toxic and controlling environment in the maternal family.

At the final Child Protection meeting, the chair commented on how lucky the couple were to have such supportive families behind them. This was so wrong that it continues to hurt me now just thinking about it. No discussion or disagreement was permitted. The paternal family was a protective factor doing everything in its power to support the couple to improve their parenting sufficiently to not need social work involvement, whereas the maternal family was exacerbating the problem, undermining the couple and being intensely hostile to any professional involvement.

Although the couple remain together with their daughter in their care, the situation is far from resolved, leaving me to continually hold a fragile dynamic together with no social work help. The wondering attitude, attentive listening and refusal to take things at face value that marks the professional curiosity model also assists in tackling disguised compliance where a family is telling you what you want to hear about acknowledgement of social work concerns and willingness to engage. That alertness and those wondering questions come in very useful here. Why is the family reluctant for me to visit the home? Why is it so difficult for me to get to see the child for whom I have concerns? Is there evidence that the birth mum has really split from her abusive partner as she says she has? Where is the evidence that drug/alcohol issues are being addressed?

This compassionate but questioning attitude can then be used to address issues of potential professional dangerousness. Am I making unsafe cultural assumptions about this family? Are they charming me into putting too much emphasis on their perspective? Is my wish to think the best of people blinding me to abuse and conflict beneath the surface? Is the child too frightened/cowed/enmeshed to open up about what things are really like for them?

By Ken Mason

Joy Salter, another person with lived experience (PWLE), a carer who also contributes to PWLE in social work education at an English higher education institution, notes that to be professionally curious, the '*the person* [practitioner] *has to know how to ask the right questions in lots of different ways*'.

> **TASK**
> - Take some time to reflect on what professional curiosity means to Ken and Joy, and what you would take forward from what they have said to inform your own practice.
> - Now list five things that come to mind about what professional curiosity means to you.
> - How would you define professional curiosity now you are on a professional course or are working with PWLE?

Involvement of people with lived experiences in safeguarding work

The involvement of PWLE in making people safe is enshrined in policy and is underpinned by best practice. In England, practitioners are guided by the Making Safeguarding Personal policy, an outcomes-focused approach that places PWLE perspectives of experiencing or being at risk of abuse and harm at the centre of what safeguarding means to them, including the outcomes they wish to achieve as the focus of intervention in adult social care (Cooper et al, 2015). In addition, the legislative frameworks underpinning safeguarding adult practice in the United Kingdom reinforce the involvement of PWLE in safeguarding adult practice to ensure that their views and outcomes are central to making people safe. Chapter 5 provides discussions on the legal and policy contexts of partnership work in adult safeguarding practice and includes the policy requirements to involve PWLE in safeguarding work.

Why is professional curiosity important in safeguarding adult practice?

The literature tells us that engagement in professional curiosity in safeguarding adult practice is important because it could save lives (Thacker et al, 2019). Serious Case Reviews (SCRs), Safeguarding Adult Reviews (SARs) and Domestic Homicide Reviews (DHRs) – these are statutory reviews carried out into the death or serious harm of an adult with care and support for learning and practice improvement – have all identified the consequences that can follow when curiosity fails to be an integral part of one's practice. The reviews identify that lack of professional curiosity led to the failure to protect individuals from abuse, neglect and harm resulting in their deaths (Muirden and Appleton, 2022; Preston-Shoot, 2017, 2023; Thacker et al, 2019, 2020). The legislative framework that guides safeguarding adult practice requires that adults who are at risk or experiencing abuse, harm and neglect are owed a duty of care and protection. Attitudes of curiosity are enshrined in safeguarding adult practice as well as professional standards (BASW, 2018; HM Inspectorate of Probation, 2022); professional curiosity is thus central to safeguarding adult practice.

It is worth acknowledging here that safeguarding adult work is characterised by complexities, ambiguities, uncertainties and indeterminacy. As well as being intellectually curious, it is important for practitioners to be socially curious. Braye et al (2017) tell us that being socially curious goes beyond having the intellectual knowledge about how something works or how a particular policy is applied. Within professional curiosity practice, having the ability to cope and manage uncertainty, ambiguity and indeterminacy are as important as having the capacity to sustain a position of certainty. Working with uncertainty, ambiguity and indeterminacy requires practitioners and those in training with the responsibility to safeguard adults to have an inquisitive mindset that goes beyond the unthinkable including going beyond agencies' policies and procedures, as practitioners need to maintain sustained relationships of trust with those at risk of or experiencing abuse, neglect and harm.

Engagement in professional curiosity is linked to notions of practising in 'safe uncertainty' and 'respectful uncertainty'. Safe uncertainty maintains a focus on safety while acknowledging that there is no certainty, and hence the desire to know more to manage the uncertainty while ensuring that the adult is safe. The notions of 'healthy scepticism' and 'respectful uncertainty' were coined by Lord Laming (2003) in the public enquiry into the death of Victoria Climbie. These notions require practitioners to be more sceptical about the information received, not taking things at face value; they need to ask respectful questions to understand what is going on in people's lives behind closed doors and in doing so save lives. In the United Kingdom and internationally, many professionals such as social workers, police, health and social care practitioners, including nurses, midwives, dentists, general practitioners, occupational therapists, physiotherapists, housing officers, support workers and those from the criminal justice system, come into contact with adults who are at risk or experiencing abuse, harm and neglect in the course of their day-to-day practice. Some of these adults are unable to protect themselves or ask for help due to illness or disabilities, while others who may be able to do so may be prevented from doing so by friends or family. Others may be unable to seek protection from harm, abuse and neglect due to shame and stigma resulting from societal norms or assumptions about abuse and neglect, and may need support from you to ensure that they are protected from abuse, harm and neglect.

In research with unpaid family carers who were at risk of or had experienced abuse by the people for whom they provided care, many reported that they were unable to report the abuse due to shame and stigma (Isham et al, 2020). Further, a review of the literature on carers who are abused by the people for whom they provide care found that safeguarding of carers is subsumed under the protection of 'adult at risk of abuse' and thus impacts the protection of carers from abuse, harm and neglect as practitioners fail to ask curious questions about carer abuse (Anka and Penhale, 2024). As practitioners, apprentices and students, you are well positioned to detect signs of abuse, harm and neglect. You have unique contact opportunities through your various roles in supporting individuals in the community and/or in institutions.

APPLYING CONCEPTS TO PRACTICE

Consider the following case study.

Case study

Imagine that you are working in a Hub. You have just been informed that B, one of the people with whom your team worked, has passed away. B was 75 years old when she died. She had a son, but they had an estranged relationship. B lived alone and did not go out. She avoided going outside as she was concerned about catching COVID-19. B therefore retreated from any form of community engagement in December 2020. Prior to B's death, nurse practitioners attending to B had reported that they had found rotting food and milk, a build-up of unwashed dishes and unmanaged faecal incontinence when they visited B and they had asked your team to contact B. In addition, your team had a phone call from the local ambulance crew reporting that B was not coping. You have been told that someone from your team had phoned B to check on her. B reassured that person that she was fine, and no further action was taken.

TASK

- What are your initial thoughts?
- How would you use professional curiosity in this case?
- What would you like to see change?
- Now read the case on which this scenario is based and consider your initial thoughts, your proposed approach and what you would like to see change: Safeguarding Adult Review – Brenda (Swindon Safeguarding Partnership, 2023).
- Make a list of what you have learnt from this case.
- How would you use what you have learnt to inform future practice?

What can we learn from Safeguarding Adult Reviews?

The case on which this case study was based is a SAR relating to Brenda that was undertaken by Swindon Safeguarding Partnership (2023) following Brenda's death in February 2021. Little was known about her life. She had multiple health and social care needs, including depression, a heart condition, kidney disease and anaemia. It was also reported that she neglected to care for herself and her environment. She had contact with her GP and weekly visits from community nurses prior to her death. A safeguarding referral was made by the community nurse and an ambulance crew to Adult Social Care Services due to difficulties with managing and maintaining her daily living activities, including personal hygiene and toileting needs. Adult Social Care Services phoned Brenda following the referral and Brenda assured them that she was okay. The SAR concluded that greater curiosity should have been shown when the Adult Social Care Team phoned Brenda and reassurances were given by Brenda that she was coping. The SAR noted that Brenda's presentation and statements were taken at face value without sufficient investigation.

The legislative framework underpinning safeguarding adult practice in England stipulates that the purpose of SAR is for learning and not to proportion blame. It is not uncommon to start with limited information. Engagement in professionally curious practice allows practitioners to persist through using empathic curiosity. Williams and Chisholm (2018, p 201) point out that professional curiosity *'involves listening to the undercurrents in the conversation and identifying what could be cries for help'*. Factors such as having comorbidities (multiple different illnesses and disabilities) impact personal lives and the ability to adequately undertake self-care. We are usually unable to take full care for ourselves and our environment when we are unwell. Writing from nursing perspectives, Procter and Wilson (2018, p 187) point out that professional curiosity compels practitioners *'to look beyond the current state and behaviours of those in* [their] *care so that a more complete "picture" of the issues and circumstances are fully understood'*. Professional curiosity practice is based on evidence-gathering and evidence-based practice. Being professionally curious requires practitioners to show concerned curiosity, which means showing genuine interest in the person with whom they work. It is about asking respectful questions about all possible signs of abuse, neglect and harm. It is also about knowing the personal histories of people, including who is and is not involved in the person's life. Being professionally curious allows the opportunity to ask courageous questions to find out what is going in the person's life. It also entails being courageous to challenge in a respectful way, checking, reflecting and not taking things at face value about what others tell you but corroborating the information received from the individual, families, friends, carers and other practitioners, and using this evidence base to inform decisions.

It is quite possible that what *appears* to be the case is likely to shift and change as new information emerges. In such situations the literature suggests that we should continue to ask questions, ask again, listen, clarify, *'know, act, ask again, recognize and understand'* as you gather the information needed to minimise the risk of abuse, harm and neglect (Freire 1998, p 80). Importantly, using empathic curiosity requires understanding of risk and what safeguarding means from the perspectives of others. Barnett (2019) asks an interesting question in her text on what safeguarding means to people. In her work, she heard different views on what it meant to people. In safeguarding adults practice, using professional curiosity enabled practitioners and those entering safeguarding adult work to gain a fuller understanding of what safeguarding means to the person at risk of experiencing abuse and neglect. This may involve seeking and clarifying information from or about the person at risk or experiencing risk of abuse and harm, from carers and families as well as from the professionals that surround the person needing protection. It is important too to remember that practitioners have a legal mandate to be professionally curious. Central to our legal mandate to being professionally curious is Article 2 of the *Human Rights Act 1998*, which is concerned with the right to life. Starns (2019) provides detailed discussions about the UK approach to safeguarding adults, including the legal duties owed to those experiencing and or at risk of harm, abuse and neglect. We encourage you to look at it. As well as analysing presenting evidence for accuracy, you need to consider changing contexts in terms of timelines of information and the evidence gathered, and the need to respond to change in a holistic way. Being professionally curious is about asking the unthinkable and seeking different perspectives. For more reading on different categories and signs of abuse see Starns' (2019) text *Safeguarding Adults Together Under the Care Act 2014: A Multi-agency Practice Guide*. Below, we explore the core skills and attributes required for professional curiosity practice in safeguarding work.

APPLYING CONCEPTS TO PRACTICE

Scenario

Imagine that you are at a busy post office, the self-checkout is out of order and you are in a long queue. The person immediately ahead of you is engaged in a conversation with another person who is also in the queue, in front of them. By the end of the queuing, the other person has told the person in front of you all about their challenging childhood and a messy divorce that they are going through and the person immediately in front of you has offered comfort. When leaving the post office, you notice that the person who had shared their story has left behind a scarf. You run to catch the person who was immediately in front of you to let them know their friend has left their scarf behind only to find out that they are not friends – they actually just met for the first time at the post office.

TASK

- Reflect on what you have learnt about yourself. What skills did you use and why might this be important in professional curiosity practice. You could also use the four different types of curiosity as a guide.

In undertaking this task, you might have listed a number of your skills and attributes, including observation, listening and thinking, tolerance, persistence, kindness and thoughtfulness. These are all very important skills in professional curiosity practice. Central to safeguarding work is protecting a person's rights to live in safety and free from abuse and neglect. This involves the skills needed to gather information about risk of harm, abuse and neglect from the individual at risk of or experiencing abuse, harm or neglect, family and carers, and other practitioners; it also includes emotional and legal literacy so one knows when to act. Table 1.3 presents a summary of the core skills and attributes required for professional curiosity practice in safeguarding adults. We explore the core skills and attributes required in more depth and with case examples in Chapter 6.

Table 1.3 A summary of core skills, abilities and attributes required for professional curiosity practice in safeguarding adults

- Effective communication skills (eg active listening, the ability to think, reflect, effectively ask questions to clarify thoughts, the ability to deal with silence and difficult emotions; the ability to ask questions without being intrusive)
- A zeal to explore
- Observation skills
- Questioning skills (eg open, probing, clarifying skills, required to identify and gather evidence from a range of sources)
- Risk-assessment skills
- Self-awareness (including an awareness of intersectional factors and impact)
- Sense-making and professional judgement
- Reflexivity, critical and analytical thinking which enables hypothesis testing and fosters curiosity
- An intuitive awareness that something is not right, which prompts a need to unpick those gut feelings
- Intuition of incoherence
- Diagnostic reasoning and investigation skills
- Courage needed to ask difficult courageous questions
- Ability to ask wondering questions
- Cultural competence and cultural humility
- Accountability
- Recognition of the need for other practitioners' involvement
- The ability to handle delicate situations
- Trust
- Empathy and compassion skills
- Genuineness
- Openness (eg the ability to build relationship of trust)
- Honesty about what one can and cannot do
- Creativity

- Empathy including perspective talk (eg the ability to understand others' perspectives on risk in what safeguarding means to them)
- Emotional intelligence (eg the ability to make emotionally informed judgements and analytical evaluation)
- Resilience
- Persistence – the ability to persist in the face of setbacks
- Attentiveness
- Stress tolerance
- Effective decision-making skills
- The ability to weigh up and synthesise information.
- Advocacy
- Inquisition and exploratory skills
- Skills and ability to notice simple things, including non-verbal clues

Evidence supporting this summary can be found in HM Inspectorate of Probation (2022); Muirden and Appleton (2022); Thacker et al (2019, 2020); Williams and Chisholm (2018).

The role of organisations in promoting professional curiosity

While most conceptualisations of professional curiosity in the practice literature have focused on individual practitioners' skills, attributes and behaviour, analysis of SARs and research highlights the important role that organisations such as local authorities, the National Health Service (NHS), police, schools, prisons and probation, housing, non-for-profit community-based organisations and charities have in supporting practitioners who participate in professional curiosity work (Preston-Shoot, 2017; 2023; Thacker et al, 2020). Muirden and Appleton (2022) remind us that the notion of professional curiosity goes beyond skills and attributes required of frontline practitioners in direct contact with those owed the duty of care of protection from abuse and neglect. The authors note that professional curiosity requires a whole-system approach, and should include *'empathic organisations, that value staff contributions and place* [people who use services] *best interests at the forefront of service development'* (Muirden and Appleton, 2022, p 3885). Like Muirden and Appleton (2022), Maynard and Cramphorn (2021) call on organisations to provide consistent support to practitioners who participate in professional curiosity practice due to the emotional labour of work. This is echoed by Thacker et al (2020), who called on strategic leaders in safeguarding adult practice to address structural barriers to professional curiosity practice. These barriers include a lack of supervision, excessive workload, the impact of new ways working, remote working and back-to-back Zoom meetings that do not allow time to reflect. (We provide more detailed discussions on barriers and facilitators to professional curiosity in Chapters 2 and 3.) Procter and Wilson (2018) note that engagement in professional curiosity practice at the organisational level includes data comprehension and analytical techniques – for example, using data to prioritise prevention. This centres on the ability of organisations and institutions to use personal data with people's consent to determine how issues such as comorbidities, psychological and emotional well-being, caring responsibilities, social, environmental and socio-economic factors impact people's lives to inform decisions about risk and risk-enablement strategies that are co-created with those owed the duty of care of protection and abuse and their families. Such data-generation activities can also be used to determine people's engagement with community services and care provision or the lack of it, including both formal and informal support.

Conclusion

This chapter has focused on the concepts of curiosity and professional curiosity. It examined why professional curiosity is important in safeguarding adult practice. It also looked at the core skills and attributes required for professional curiosity practice in safeguarding adult work and organisations' responsibilities for supporting practitioners who are engaged in professional curiosity practice. It is hoped that you will use the knowledge gained from reading this chapter to work to inform engagement in professional curiosity practice and in partnership with people who are at risk of or experiencing abuse, harm and neglect, their families and carers, and with other professionals in protecting their human rights to live in safety, free from abuse, harm and neglect.

KEY POINTS FROM THIS CHAPTER

- Curiosity enables effective risk assessment, risk-enablement and risk-management decisions to be made as well as informing creative interventions co-produced with those owed the duty of care and protection.
- Professional curiosity is central to safeguarding adult practice.
- Engagement in professional curiosity practice in safeguarding adults allows the opportunity to work in partnership within justifiable outcomes with those at risk or experiencing abuse, harm and neglect, families, carers and practitioners surrounding the individual to protect and prevent deaths from abuse, harm and neglect.

→

- Practitioners engaged in safeguarding adult practice are uniquely placed to use professional curiosity to work in collaboration with those at risk of or experiencing abuse, harm and neglect, their families and with other practitioners who surround those at risk of harm.
- You demonstrate professional curiosity by showing a genuine desire to know, showing interest in people as individuals, engaging in empathetic courageous conversations, asking respectful questions about all possible signs of abuse and neglect, listening, reflecting, clarifying, exploring, examining, critically evaluating and analysing evidence gathered from different perspectives.

Further reading

HM Inspectorate of Probation (2022) *Practitioner: Professional Curiosity Insights guide*. Manchester: HM Inspectorate of Probation. [online] Available at: www.justiceinspectorates.gov.uk/hmiprobation.

A useful and accessible practice guide for practitioners and managers in probation. Explores what professional curiosity is, also provides insight about the barriers and facilitators of professional curiosity.

Kashdan, T B Stiksma, M C, Disabato, D J, McKnight, P E, Bekier, J, Kaji, J and Lazarus, R (2018) The Five-Dimensional Curiosity Scale: Capturing the Bandwidth of Curiosity and Identifying Four Unique Subgroups of Curious People. *Journal of Research in Personality*, 73: 130–49.

Offers valuable insights into different dimensions of curiosity.

Starns, B (2019) *Safeguarding Adults Together Under the Care Act 2014: A Multi-agency Practice Guide*. St Albans: Critical Publishing.

An accessible book on safeguarding adults under the Care Act 2014 in multi-professional context.

Thacker, H, Anka, A and Penhale, B (2019) Could Curiosity Save Lives? An Exploration into the Value of Employing Professional Curiosity and Partnership Work in Safeguarding Adults Under the *Care Act 2014*. *Journal of Adult Protection*, 21(5): 252–67.

Examines the barriers and facilitators of professional curiosity and partnership work in safeguarding adults drawing from analysis of SARs.

2 Barriers to professional curiosity in safeguarding adults

CHAPTER OBJECTIVES

By the end of this chapter, you should be able to:

- know some of the key barriers to professional curiosity;
- identify a range of barriers which may obstruct your use of professional curiosity in daily practice and develop strategies to address these;
- understand the reasons why these barriers may be present;
- place these barriers to professional curiosity in a wider systems context.

Introduction

The chapter explores barriers to effective professional curiosity in safeguarding adults. It draws from the broad literature, research and lessons to be learnt from practice, SARs and CSPRs. As described in Chapter 1, professional curiosity is a key practice requirement for practitioners across many service areas and professional groups, especially in social work, health and social care, education and law enforcement. More recently, professional curiosity has increasingly been considered within an adult safeguarding context (Thacker et al, 2020). It is embedded in safeguarding adult policies and law. Professional curiosity is a well-established term across safeguarding networks, promoted by various safeguarding adult boards and child safeguarding partnerships in briefing documents. Yet repeated safeguarding reviews identify a lack of 'professional curiosity' and insufficient 'challenge' on the part of practitioners as the cause of common and recurring shortcomings, both for children (Dickens et al, 2023) and adults (Thacker et al, 2019, 2020), as well as in other practice areas, including probation (Phillips et al, 2022) and education (Cramphorn and Maynard, 2023). This concurs with a recent analysis of 652 Safeguarding Adults Reviews (SARs), completed between April 2019 and March 2023, and supported with returns from all 136 safeguarding adult boards in England (Preston-Shoot et al, 2024). From the 652 reviews detailing practice shortcomings in direct work with the person, absence of professional curiosity was highlighted in 100 of these SARs (44 per cent), the fifth highest out of a total of 27 areas identified. Alongside the quantitative data analysis of all 652 SARs, a separate report focused on the in-depth, detailed learning identified in a smaller, stratified sample (229 SARs) Preston-Shoot et al (2024). This qualitative analysis provides valuable insights into the barriers practitioners can experience to carry out professionally curious practice. From this analysis, professional curiosity was the single key omission in practice, noted in multiple SARs. In direct work with individuals, only 3 per cent of reviews in the qualitative analysis noted positive practice relating to professional curiosity (Preston-Shoot et al, 2024).

The analysis identified examples from SARs where there were missed opportunities to understand reluctance to engage with services, risk assessment, carer needs, rapidly escalating health needs, repeated Accident and Emergency (A&E) attendance and not seeking information about what might be happening – for example, in family relationships or when the adult 'dropped out of sight' (Preston-Shoot et al, 2024). There was also evidence of a lack of challenge, accepting accounts at face value and missed opportunities to explore what might lie behind presenting problems. Preston-Shoot et al (2024, p 41) summarise these shortcomings:

> *Attention tended to be focused on what was presented rather than seeking out what was not, and upon the presenting problem rather than on asking questions that could reveal its causes. Practitioners sometimes relied on self-reports by the individual, for example that they were taking their medication, in the face of evidence that they were most probably not. In one case, practitioners failed to see beyond self-soiling behaviours that could have been forms of communication about underlying distress, merely accepting that 'this is her'.*

In some cases, as in the example noted below, the absence of professional curiosity had a tangible impact on intervention, with care hours being cut because they were not being used. Preston-Shoot et al (2024, p 41) reported that

> *there was a lack of curiosity demonstrated by the reviewing social worker, which led to a significant reduction in X's hours of care. X's whole situation and history were not accounted for in this review, nor the reasons why she was not utilising the part of her care package that would help her to access the community.*

The authors argue that professional curiosity performs a critical practice role as one of the skills best tailored to engaging, building rapport and developing person-centred relationships (Preston-Shoot et al, 2024). It is also sometimes an important gateway to identifying abuse and neglect, probing below the surface of appearances to reveal a safeguarding need. Dickens et al (2023, p 2) note that the reasons for this lack of professional curiosity remain poorly understood and that, '*without interrogating why, when and in what circumstances it becomes more difficult for professionals to remain open, curious and appropriately challenging*'.

Other authors have identified the use of '*curious or courageous questions*' to involve and engage people themselves in safeguarding. Here, curiosity is seen as the challenge needed in *situations where there are assumptions about why someone is in a safeguarding situation, rather than focusing on the problems they face as a result, can individualise or pathologise the issues as well as the solutions.*

(Hafford-Letchfield and Carr, 2017, p 99)

Being professionally curious, argue Hafford-Letchfield and Carr (2017), provides the opportunity to support a more outcome-focused and person-centred approach to practice. What follows explores some of the key barriers to professional curiosity.

Barriers to professional curiosity

Barriers to professional curiosity can be experienced by people working in a wide range of roles across different sectors and in a range of circumstances, including the statutory, voluntary and community sectors. In setting out the barriers to professional curiosity, Thacker et al (2019) identified three groupings: '*case dynamics*', '*professional issues*' and '*organisational issues*'. Phillips et al (2024) used an alternative approach to delineate barriers: *structural*', '*relational*' and '*emotional*'. This chapter has used a blend of these groups to explore the barriers to professional curiosity under the following headings (see Table 2.1):

- Personal issues (emotional);
- Case dynamics (relational);
- Organisational (structural);
- Systematic (socio-systemic).

Table 2.1 The barriers to professional curiosity practice in safeguarding adults

Grouping	Factors
Personal issues (personal level)	Emotional exhaustion and burnout
	Compassion fatigue
	Secondary trauma
	Personal bias and assumptions
	Cognitive bias
	Lack of cultural curiosity
	Lack of confidence
	Fear of reaction
	Fear of making mistakes

Grouping	Factors
Case dynamics	Limited knowledge base
	Disguised compliance
	Rule of optimism/minimising risk
	Normalisation
	'Knowing but not knowing'
	Professional deference
Organisational issues	Bureaucratic processes
	Inadequate supervision
	Resource constraints
	Increasing workload pressures
	High workload and lack of time
	Organisational culture
	Insufficient training and development)
Systemic issues	Climate of austerity
	Increasing demand on services
	Policy and legislative context
	Societal attitudes/stigma
	Overarching political/cultural context

It is worth pointing out that while these groups have been used to organise the material, clear crossover and links exist between the topics discussed. For example, barriers presented by emotional exhaustion and burnout sit at a personal level for practitioners but are often caused by organisational and wider systematic issues.

APPLYING CONCEPTS TO PRACTICE

Case study

Jo is a social worker. She is visiting Pat, a 73 year-old woman referred by her GP. Jo's neighbour reported that she wasn't coping at home. The neighbour said Pat's house was full of clutter and she hadn't been getting out of bed. Jo asked whether Pat's health had been assessed, but the GP said, 'It's a social problem.' Jo had a feeling the GP hadn't seen Pat but didn't like to challenge a doctor and the GP sounded very confident. Jo is exhausted as she sets off to visit Pat, who she's never met before. She's covering for her colleague Chris, who's off sick, and she's been bombarded by calls and emergencies all week. She knocks quietly on the door, leaves it for five seconds and turns to go, telling herself that Pat must be out and she can leave with a clear conscience as she did her best to visit.

Just as Jo reaches the gate, a clipped, aggressive-sounding male voice shouts, 'Who is it?' Jo feels she must return to the house and calls out that it's Jo from adult social care. The door is opened by a diminutive man wearing a suit who looks very irritated. The man says he is Pat's son, Martin. Jo wishes she'd made time to read Pat's record before she set off from the office; she didn't know Pat had a son. Jo feels uncomfortable. Martin is hostile towards her, saying, 'I thought you lot were leaving us alone now Chris has left.' Jo picks her way through a small path that has formed through a large amount of clutter and enters Pat's bedroom. There is a strong smell of urine. Jo remembers that Chris (her colleague) always came back from visiting Pat saying the house smelt really bad. Jo asks Martin how Pat is getting on. Martin says they're fine and that he's phoned up about getting some grab rails for Pat as the last social worker Chris said she would do, but there is no sign that she has actually done so. Jo thinks, 'What a relief; that's one less thing for me to do.' Martin is becoming agitated and says he's getting rather tired of social workers sniffing about when he's doing his best to look after his mum.

Jo feels intimidated and decides to leave. She gets up to say goodbye to Pat, who shrinks back a little as she approaches. She notices that Pat has some purple bruises on her arm. 'Older people often lose their balance and knock into things,' she thinks. Jo leaves quickly and feels relief to be out of the house, but her sense of unease lingers. She gives her manager a ring and leaves a message asking for a call back. At 6pm she hasn't heard back, so she pours herself a glass of wine and finally starts to feel better. The following day, Jo is allocated another three adults to assess, so decides to close Pat's case. Pat has her son to support her, and she has always been fine before so she'll be fine this time too. Three months later, the police are called by Pat's neighbour, who heard shouting in the house. Pat has been murdered by her son. The county community safety partnership opens a domestic homicide review.

TASK

- Drawing from Table 2.1 (barriers to professional curiosity), identify key barriers to professional curiosity raised in this case study.
- What curious questions would you ask in this context?

- Now write a short reflective piece about how you are feeling about the outcome of this case and share it with a trusted colleague who can provide some emotional support if needed.
- Progressing forward, make a list of what you could do differently.

We return to this case study in Chapter 3 when we consider enablers of professional curiosity.

What follows explores potential barriers to professional curiosity, starting with those relating to personal issues.

Barriers to professional curiosity: personal issues

Any consideration of what might inhibit the use of professional curiosity by a practitioner must first and foremost acknowledge the personal impact on that individual. This may include, for example, their perceived ability to cope in their job role, motivations and perception of personal responsibility ('this is not my job'). Other factors include the potential impact of the environment in which practice happens (is it safe enough to facilitate further disclosure?) and relationships (with both the people they support and the people with whom they work).

Emotional exhaustion and burnout

Various advantageous personality traits, attitudes, behaviours and skills have been identified that support the use of professional curiosity (Thacker et al, 2020), but it requires personal strength, tenacity and determination to sustain oneself when faced with adversity. Emotional exhaustion and burnout, common in high-stress professions such as healthcare and social work, can diminish the energy and motivation required for professional curiosity. Professional curiosity requires a high degree of what Phillips et al (2024) call 'surface acting', which in turn is linked to burnout. Research demonstrates that due to increased pressures on services, particularly during and after the COVID-19 pandemic, practitioners who are feeling overwhelmed with work and who are mentally and emotionally depleted are less likely to engage deeply with their cases or make a curious enquiry (Lluch et al, 2022; Spányik et al, 2023). Phillips et al (2024) argue that organisations should be mindful of the emotional toll of work in health and human service professions, especially when workloads are high, because burnout tends to have its roots in poor work environments rather than individuals. The literature identifies that high caseload pressures impact a person's ability to ask curious questions. Reder et al (1993), cited by Burton and Revell (2018), note that individuals with high caseloads are more likely to step back from asking a question, knowing that if they ask it, they will have to be prepared to respond to the answer and it may well create more work. When this happens, we take in what is happening around us with one part of our mind, but with another we fail to analyse what we have seen (Burton and Revell, 2018).

Compassion fatigue

Another key barrier to professional curiosity is compassion fatigue, which relates to feeling overwhelmed by the suffering of others and then impacts one's ability to care. Research shows that an individual's human compassion response often weakens with repeated exposure to suffering. The literature suggests that continuous exposure to traumatic stories and high-stress environments can lead to compassion fatigue in those working in human services professions – for example, in healthcare (Garnett et al, 2023) and social work (Kinman and Grant, 2020). Compassion fatigue is often used interchangeably in the literature with vicarious traumatisation, secondary traumatic stress and empathy-based stress. Cocker and Joss (2016) point out that compassion fatigue is caused by stress resulting from exposure to traumatic personal stories and or traumatic environments. In the nursing literature, compassion fatigue has been linked to *'the stress accumulated within nurses over time due to their provision of prolonged care, support, and assistance to others, leading to emotional, physiological, and psychological exhaustion'* (Chu, 2024, p 20). Research demonstrates that compassion fatigue impacts decision-making and our ability to care and provide appropriate support (Filipponi et al, 2024; Sabanciogullari et al, 2021). Safeguarding work is complex, and it can be emotionally distressing to repeatedly listen to distressing and traumatic stories of those who are at risk of or experiencing abuse, harm and neglect. Like safeguarding children's work, work in safeguarding adults has an emotional dimension, which can be distressing, stressful, emotionally draining and upsetting. Burton and Revell (2018, p 1515) note that,

> on an individual level, workers are forced to confront the possibility of harm to children [adults] and, along with this, the myriad personal feelings that they may experience, generating tension or a state of cognitive dissonance by managing or holding different, conflicting perspectives.

Compassion fatigue can reduce a practitioner's ability and willingness to engage deeply with people who use services and their situations, and this can consequently dent professional curiosity. Warning signs of compassion fatigue include emotional disconnectedness, loss of interests, reduced feeling of empathy and sensitivity, anxiety, irritability, indifference, inability to make decisions and burnout (Chu, 2024; Filipponi et al, 2024).

Secondary trauma

Like compassion fatigue, exposure to the traumatic experience of others and/or an environment can lead to secondary trauma. For example, where professionals and other visitors to health, care or home settings repeatedly witness situations of neglect, poor care or multiple safeguarding concerns, it can lead to desensitisation, normalisation, detachment, stress, anxiety and burnout. The ensuing loss of empathy, engagement and inevitably curiosity will limit the effectiveness of the protection or prevention of harm to children or adults at risk.

The SAR into the deaths of Joanna, Jon and Ben in a private hospital setting commissioned by Norfolk Safeguarding Adults Board (NSAB, 2021) gives two examples of secondary trauma. First, the review noted the very high levels of 'challenging behaviour' by the patients, evidenced through incident forms, but also that professionals often failed to question, to be curious about what sat behind the behaviour – failing to consider why the behaviour was happening. In that case, some very clear antecedents were identified. These included abusive and neglectful care, a lack of meaningful activity, a lack of routine, failure to recognise individual ways of communication, incomplete knowledge of the background, development, past traumas and the general needs of the patients (Norfolk Safeguarding Adults Board, 2021).

Second, this SAR demonstrates how a specific trauma experienced by those providing direct care (here staff were repeatedly subjected to racial abuse by the adults they were supporting) can give rise to an abusive and neglectful culture. In most settings, organisations will have a 'zero tolerance' approach to abuse of staff. However, when those being abusive have limited or no meaningful control over their words or behaviour because of mental health needs or cognitive difficulties, there are very limited sanctions available. Organisations are mandated with statutory responsibility to provide care or treatment; they also have statutory responsibility to provide a safe working environment for their staff. The SAR found that in the hospital where Joanna, Jon and Ben were patients, abuse of staff had become normalised. Unsupported staff became increasingly detached in their caring roles, leading to reciprocal abuse and neglect of the patients living there. It is important to seek support when the work environment does not support respectful and safe practice. Drawing from the 'oxygen mask theory', from airline safety protocols, you can take the following basic steps to effect change. The 'oxygen mask theory' recognises that you first need to fit your own 'oxygen mask' or you will not be well enough or be able to help others with theirs.

Secondary trauma: 'Fitting your own oxygen mask'

Here are some practice pointers from the Norfolk Safeguarding Adults Board (2023) seven-minute briefing on trauma.

- Seek support/talk to your manager; make use of reflective practice/supervision (if you have it).
- Be honest about how you are feeling; be non-judgemental towards others who share their feelings; remember, your own perspective is unique, as are those of the people around you.
- Understand the strength in recognising your needs early and acting – think about what triggers your own 'fight/flight/freeze/flop/friend' responses – what does that look like for you, what can you do to disrupt that instinctive response?
- Use preventative strategies – self-care, breathing exercises, physical exercise, time out.

- Where a situation has affected several people, think about having a peer or team debrief – a chance for all of you to get together and reflect on what has happened, to unpick it and how it made each of you feel, and to work out how to move forward.

Personal bias and assumptions

Humans are hard-wired to make intuitive decisions about other people and we do this many times every day. These intuitive unconscious judgements affect our attitudes and behaviours, and help us to determine whether someone might be friendly or hostile. Using a range of information – visual, verbal and behavioural – we go through a process of rapid categorisation that is both natural and necessary for day-to-day functioning. For instance, we instantly categorise individuals by age, gender, ethnicity, social background, sexual orientation or education.

While this evolutionary system saves us time and effort processing information about people (and has kept us alive as a species), the clear disadvantage is that we can make assumptions about people and take action based on those assumptions and biases. This results in a tendency to rely on stereotypes, *even if we don't consciously believe in them* – shifting us from danger detectors to social labelling and stereotyping that leads to high levels of prejudice and discrimination. For example, the use of the 'myth of lifestyle choice' in self-neglect situations reduces receptiveness to other possible explanations. Professional curiosity requires you to check and challenge your personal biases. Bias and assumptions have implications for how you may or may not use professional curiosity in safeguarding practice. Unconscious biases are seen to lead practitioners to:

- accept the first explanation, as the only possible explanation;
- be rigid about what you believe to be true;
- only select information which confirms the question at hand and your belief about this.

REFLECTIVE QUESTION

- Take up to ten minutes to reflect and make notes on your personal biases and assumptions and consider their implications for practice.

Cognitive bias

Cognitive biases, such as confirmation bias, relate to the tendency to search for or interpret information in a way that confirms one's preconceptions. When this happens, practitioners often seek information that confirms their pre-existing beliefs, overlooking contradictory evidence that might be crucial for a thorough and objective assessment. Similarly, anchoring bias relates to the reliance on the first piece of information encountered. Other examples of cognitive bias include adultification bias. Citing Davis and Marsh (2020), Davis (2022, p 5) notes that adultification bias occurs *'when notions of innocence and vulnerability are not afforded to certain children'*. This potentially affects curiosity and effective agency responses. For more reading on adultification bias, see Wirral Safeguarding Children Partnership (2022) (Child Q), where children from Black, Asian and minoritised ethnic communities were perceived as more 'streetwise', less innocent and less vulnerable than other children. Also see Gloucestershire Safeguarding Children's Partnership (GSCP) (Young, 2023) (Child X). In Richmond and Wandsworth SAB's SAR of Harvey, assumptions were made across agencies that demonstrated a degree of unconscious bias in the conceptualisation and management of risk, resulting in a lack of response to incidents of interpersonal abuse (Smith and El-Kaddah, 2020). Further, in the SAR of Riley, Tameside Safeguarding Adult Board (Newman, 2023, p 25), it was noted that the review panel felt *'there was a likelihood of unconscious gender or sexuality bias in relation to perceptions of his sexual behaviour and therefore his risk of sexual exploitation'*. These biases can lead to a narrow focus and hinder the exploration of alternative perspectives.

APPLYING CONCEPTS TO PRACTICE

Case study: Camden Safeguarding Adults Partnership SAR: Hannah

Hannah, a 55 year-old woman living with Huntington's disease (HD), had a history of trauma and had received treatment for anxiety and depression. She also used alcohol and had a pattern of binge drinking, when she would often become verbally aggressive. The HD progressively affected her cognition, speech and mobility, and made her more susceptible to intoxication by alcohol. Hannah was known by health and social care services in Camden and was a frequent caller to emergency services. After a night of drinking at a local pub, she returned to her flat with a woman (Lucy) and another male. Hannah was stabbed to death that night. Lucy was convicted of her murder.

The SAR found that Hannah's frequent emergency calls following falls and reports of sexual assault (which she subsequently withdrew) were attributed to alcohol intoxication rather than possible symptoms of her HD or a trauma-related response (Smith and El-Kaddah, 2020). The report notes that *'the organisational view seemed to have settled – that Hannah was making decisions to drink alcohol, was making decisions about risk, and she could therefore protect herself from the adverse effects of both'* (Smith and El-Kaddah, 2020, p 19).

Assumptions about Hannah had been made based on her use of alcohol and risky behaviours, at the expense of her mental health needs and HD progression. Professional curiosity about Hannah's interactions with services could have identified a combination of risk factors for exploitation and abuse and helped to develop protective risk plans to support her.

A lack of cultural curiosity

Cultural curiosity refers to the desire to learn about other people's cultures, to understand how a person's culture impacts their worldview and influences how they live their lives. Cultural curiosity makes us culturally aware and broadens our capacity to understand others' perspectives and the bases for them (Somani, 2005). A lack of cultural curiosity can lead to misunderstanding and hinder the use of professional curiosity. Practitioners who lack cultural curiosity may fail to appreciate the cultural context of their clients, leading to misunderstandings and missed opportunities for deeper enquiry. In such circumstances, interventions may be based on stereotyping or lack of awareness of how various categories of abuse are manifested in different communities, coupled with a general lack of awareness of cultural practices. Practitioners must be sensitive to differing family patterns, lifestyles and child rearing practices across different racial, ethnic and cultural groups (Okpokiri et al, 2024). The research in this area suggests that in some instances people may be reluctant to access support from a desire to keep family life private, and in many communities there is a fear of professional power (Dickens et al, 2022). It is also likely that some communities may have a poor view of support services arising from initial contact with public services (Mallorie, 2024). For further reading about the impact of the lack of cultural curiosity, see the Rochdale Borough Safeguarding Adults Board's SAR relating to Adult H (Sandiford, 2023b). The SAR noted that a lack of cultural curiosity inhibited the ability to ask curious questions (Sandiford, 2023b).

Lack of confidence

Another barrier to professional curiosity is a lack of confidence. Lacking confidence or assertiveness to ask sensitive questions may be the result of insecurity and/or self-doubt. A lack of confidence can stem from inadequate training, limited experience or previous negative feedback. A lack of self-confidence can be a significant barrier. Professionals who doubt their abilities may be less likely to question existing practices or seek deeper understanding, fearing that they might appear incompetent or ignorant. They may hesitate to ask probing questions or challenge information provided by clients, colleagues or supervisors because they do not feel confident to deal with the response to the question. A lack of confidence is frequently attributed to inadequate initial training and limited opportunities for continuous professional development.

Fear of the reaction

We are less likely to ask questions – particularly if those questions are perceived as probing or challenging in some way – if the likely response is known to be hostile and angry. Violence against health and social care staff is a well-documented, real and daily threat (Tuominen et al, 2023). Evidence shows that anxiety inhibits curiosity (Kashdan et al, 2018). Disagreements or aggression from families or others towards practitioners can erode the confidence needed to keep a focus on the concern in question, diverting meetings away from the topics the professional wants to explore in more depth.

> ### APPLYING CONCEPTS TO PRACTICE
> #### Case study
> Stephen (aged 59) had been a long-term patient at a neurological centre, following head injuries (Solihull SAB, 2018). When he was diagnosed with terminal cancer, he was discharged to his own flat with 24/7 2:1 care, to be near his family for his final remaining days (in the event, he lived for 14 months). Stephen choked to death on food while alone in his flat. He had previously choked on food. The SAR found that Stephen's vulnerability was perhaps disguised because he was perceived as a challenge to services. Carers reported being scared of him.

TASK
- Identify one possible barrier to professional curiosity in this case.
- What would you do to effect change?

Fear of making mistakes

Many practitioners fear making errors that could lead to negative outcomes for clients or potential career repercussions. This fear may discourage staff from asking questions or exploring new ideas.

Professional deference

Practitioners may also fear negative consequences for questioning the actions or decisions of others, especially in hierarchical environments. This is known as professional deference. Workers who have most contact with an individual are in a good position to recognise when the risks to the person are escalating. However, there can be a tendency to defer to the opinion of a 'higher status' professional, who has limited contact with the person but views the risk as less significant or serious (Thacker et al, 2019). It is a courageous act to disagree with or challenge their opinion of risk if it varies from your own. This fear can also prevent practitioners from expressing doubts or seeking further clarification.

Barriers to professional curiosity: case dynamics

Limited knowledge base

Insufficient knowledge about specific issues, such as mental health conditions, substance abuse or cultural nuances, can restrict practitioners' abilities to exercise curiosity effectively. When practitioners lack specialised knowledge, they are less likely to ask pertinent questions or recognise significant signs.

Not knowing what questions to ask and being concerned about causing offence to people can inhibit curious enquiry. We work in a complex landscape, people's lives are multi-factorial, layered and often not what they seem, and trying to unpick which might be the right questions can be a daunting prospect, even for experienced staff. Britten and Whitby (2021) have produced a useful list of questions that practitioners could use, which you might find useful.

Disguised compliance

The practice literature suggests that disguised compliance occurs when a family member or carer gives the appearance of cooperating with professionals to avoid raising suspicions, to allay concerns and ultimately to reduce professional involvement (Nicolas, 2016; NSAB 2022; Phillips et al, 2024). The practice literature suggests disguised compliance occurs when a person or family directs the focus of safeguarding concerns to criticising professionals, failing to engage with services or avoiding contact with professionals. Leigh et al's (2020) critical discourse analysis, which explored how the term has been used in social work, cautions that it should not be used uncritically. When an individual or their family erects barriers to involvement, it is important to work restoratively with them. Explore what may lie behind the barrier or resistance, explain why you are asking questions and seek clarification so they understand that your questions are well meaning and relate to their well-being and safety. You need to establish the facts and gather evidence about what is actually happening. You must focus on outcomes rather than processes, to ensure you remain person-centred.

The rule of optimism/minimising risk

Closely linked to disguised compliance is the 'rule of optimism'. This is a psychological defence mechanism used to justify inaction or a lack of professional curiosity because the nature of the potential harm is either too painful to acknowledge, or because the practitioner does not want to think their client might 'fail' (Phillips et al, 2024). Using the rule of optimism, professionals tend to rationalise away new or escalating risks, despite clear evidence to the contrary, focusing solely on the positives in a client's life. Using a self-reflective question can counterbalance this. Is progress really being made? Are intended outcomes actually being achieved?

REFLECTIVE QUESTION

- Take five minutes to think about a recent case and write any examples where you may have minimised risk or been over-optimistic about progress or potential outcomes.

Normalisation

Normalisation refers to social processes through which ideas and actions come to be seen as 'normal' and become taken for granted or 'natural' in everyday life. They stop being questioned and are not recognised or assessed as potential risks. As such, it is less likely to trigger curious questioning (Thacker et al, 2019).

A SAR carried out for Norfolk Safeguarding Adults Board (SAB) into the death of Mrs BB, an older woman living with dementia, describes how she was often found outside her house in the surrounding lanes at unusual times and was returned to her home by the police and members of the community. Other agencies were not notified as her behaviour had become 'normalised' and the cumulative risk to her was not spotted (Brabbs, 2016). Other examples can be seen in the second national SAR analysis in England. Preston-Shoot and colleagues (2024, p. 44) noted in one of the SARs that:

> X was in frequent contact with a number of agencies, making 41 separate 999 calls in the eleven months prior to his death. This, combined with his alcohol use, appeared to result in the normalisation of risk, missed opportunities to identify self-neglect and the risk of harm from others and the inability to see him as a whole person or to recognise how vulnerable and isolated he was.

Knowing but not knowing

Thacker et al (2019) note that knowing but not knowing relates to having a sense that something is not right but not knowing exactly what that is, which means it can be difficult to fully grasp the problem, make appropriate plans and take relevant action. The theme 'knowing but not knowing' was identified by Ferguson (2017), cited in Burton and Revell (2018, p 1516), to explain the complex processes at work in the Victoria Climbie case. They note:

> [Professionals] became bystanders to an appalling atrocity. They knew but they didn't know what was happening to Victoria and did nothing ... This is another example of the avoidant behaviour professionals engage in when faced with intolerable feelings stirred up by having to think the unthinkable about what may have been done to a child.

Barriers to professional curiosity: organisational issues

Bureaucratic processes

Complex and cumbersome bureaucratic processes can stifle professional curiosity. Strict adherence to organisational protocols (a 'just following instructions' mentality) prevents the use of professional judgement and discourages exploratory questioning. The more organisational policies and procedures explicitly allow for professional discretion and flexibility, the more freedom there is for professionals to exercise curiosity and judgement in their work.

Inadequate supervision

Thacker et al (2020) note that high-quality supervision provides access to a safe space for exploring complex safeguarding cases, which is essential for aiding reflective practice and developing professional curiosity. Without opportunities for reflection, to ask questions and to receive challenges about what is happening in a particular case during supervision, any assumptions made by a practitioner can remain fixed. Wilkins' (2024) framework for supervisors (and organisations) includes 'exploring multiple perspectives' – something that is enabled through use of professional curiosity. Inadequate supervision is therefore a significant barrier to professionally curious practice, yet many practitioners report that their supervision is either infrequent or lacks depth. Revell and Burton (2016) also note that ensuring compliance with standards and promoting the positive well-being of individual practitioners in supervision can create complex relational dynamics. They propose that the rule of optimism (see above) may be transposed onto the supervisory relationship and, as in frontline practice, stifle effective use of professional curiosity. Supervisors should be trained to support practitioners in developing their investigative skills and professional curiosity.

Resource constraints

Increasing workload pressures

The health and social care system continues to face well-documented pressures. Austerity measures, funding pressures and analysis of SARs demonstrate that a lack of resources have significantly impacted practice (Bottery and Mallorie, 2024; Care Quality Commission, 2024; Preston-Shoot et al, 2024). Increased workload and lack of resources significantly impact professional curiosity. In such a context, there may be a tendency (whether consciously or otherwise) to create an environment that prevents further disclosure. High caseloads and administrative burdens can leave practitioners with insufficient time to engage deeply with each case. Time pressures can lead to superficial assessments and hinder thorough investigation and assessment. Limited resources, including frequent changes in practitioners, are substantial barriers to professional curiosity. Repeatedly 'starting again' can hinder professional curiosity (Thacker et al, 2019). High turnover of social workers has been shown to impact the ability to develop relationships over time with clients/service users. Financial constraints can limit access to training, supervision, and other resources that support the development of professional curiosity. Organisations may struggle to provide the necessary support for their staff to engage in thorough and reflective practice. Thacker et al (2019, 2020) noted that education and training programmes that prioritise technical skills over soft skills, such as communication, empathy and critical thinking, may leave professionals ill-equipped to engage in professional curiosity. A balanced approach is essential for fostering inquisitive mindsets.

> **APPLYING CONCEPTS TO PRACTICE**
>
> ### Case study
>
> The SAR of Philip commissioned by City and Hackney Safeguarding Adults Board illustrates the impact of resource constraints (Williams and Bateman, 2022). Philip was evicted from the family home after his wife reported his emotionally and physically abusive behaviour and alcohol misuse. A week later, a family member contacted the children's social worker about them being left in Philip's care and raised concerns about historic offences. Shortly afterwards, Philip attempted suicide and was informally admitted to hospital. He was subsequently placed in B&B accommodation, while returning to hospital every day for support. After disclosing serious historic offences to the police, he was given the opportunity to seek legal advice before a formal interview. He was found dead in his room four days later.
>
> An overarching theme of the SAR was pressure on the system because of high levels of need and professionals having to prioritise caseloads in terms of support and the assumptions made about reduced follow-ups.

TASK

- Working with a colleague, take five minutes to identify what support, if any, is available in your local authority for families that may be experiencing similar difficulties.

High workload and lack of time

Phillips et al (2024) have identified that excessive workloads and time pressures contribute to reduced professional curiosity. A study using online focus groups emphasised the obstacles to professional curiosity posed by heavy workloads, high staff turnover and sickness rates (Dickens et al, 2023). One view was that '*staff know what they should be doing, but can't*' (Dickens et al, 2022, p113). Time pressure often leads to rushed assessments and missed critical details. Practitioners under constant pressure to manage numerous cases often prioritise immediate tasks over thorough investigation. A combination of lack of time, pressure of workloads and priority given to short-term and time-limited involvement over relationship-based practice restricts the space for professional curiosity to operate, or even at times to develop. High caseloads and time pressures can lead to burnout, limiting the mental and emotional energy available for practitioners to exercise curiosity and thorough investigation. In addition, some newly qualified, inexperienced workers might not be confident about what they should be doing even if they knew about it from their training.

Organisational culture

If practitioners do not feel safe to ask questions and express doubts without fear of reprisal, it does not foster professional curiosity across an organisation. The organisational context of proceduralisation (Dickens et al, 2023) may prioritise paperwork over in-depth client engagement, acting as a brake on professional curiosity (Burton and Revell, 2018). Good guidance and support for new staff are essential (Dickens et al, 2023). As Dickens et al (2023, p 6) note,

> *developing the necessary skills and providing the right support requires an understanding of the complex psychological, practical and organisational factors that make this difficult. Setting curiosity and challenge within wider frames of communication and courage could be a productive route.*

Insufficient training and development

Insufficient in-service training leads to an information gap and hinders professional curiosity. Professionals who have not been taught how to effectively question assumptions, think critically, use cultural curiosity, gather information and analyse data from different perspectives may struggle to apply these skills in their safeguarding work. Although some local Safeguarding Adults Boards (SABs) have attempted to address these training gaps, which have been highlighted in numerous SARs, they are somewhat ad hoc, with a fallback position relying on practitioners to 'pick it up' along the way. An integrative review of health and social care practitioners' experiences of using professional curiosity in child protection practice carried out by Muirden and Appleton (2022) concludes that practitioners need this expertise and that their organisations (including multi-agency partnerships and professional bodies) should be held accountable. The authors urged organisations to consider

> *whether their mandatory training and competency frameworks fully encompass the high-level communication skills required [for professional curiosity], including the building of empathic relationships, to promote an effective workforce. Likewise, communication skills training needs to be woven throughout health and social care professional practice courses, to continually build and strengthen the confidence and competence of practitioners working within a very challenging yet also very rewarding area of practice.*
>
> (Muirden and Appleton, 2022, p e3909)

A lack of ongoing opportunities for continuing professional development can hinder professional curiosity. Without regular training updates and exposure to new ideas, professionals may become stagnant in their thinking and practices.

> **REFLECTIVE QUESTIONS**
> - Does your organisation specifically train its workforce in how to be curious?
> - Work with a colleague, take five minutes and develop a training programme on professional curiosity for colleagues in your team. What specific issues would you like to explore?

Barriers to professional curiosity: systemic factors

Climate of austerity

The impact of austerity has been highlighted by Bateman (2018) and in the second national SAR analysis in England (Preston-Shoot et al, 2024). Here, analysis of SARs identified that austerity had resulted in demand management and reduced professional curiosity. Barriers to professional curiosity have been set out above at the personal, professional and organisational levels. However, the context in which practitioners work, and in which organisations operate and deliver services, is located at the macro-level. It could be argued that barriers at these other levels flow from the systemic macro-level policy context. This policy arena is described as neoliberal, in which *'risks are seen to be situated in the individual and where responsibility for managing that risk falls to individual practitioners and service use'* (Kemshall, 2002, cited in Phillips et al, 2024, p 324). It is understandable that practitioners might be cautious about the requirement for curiosity in their practice. When things go wrong (a person experiences abuse or harm or even dies) there is potentially significant media and public attention that is more likely to place responsibility with the individual practitioner, without considering the context of practice. For Phillips et al (2024), this individualising and individualised approach within policy is problematic because it fails to account for structural issues and factors that can inhibit professional curiosity. Phillips et al (2024) argue that rising demands, coupled with resource limitations and a reduced workforce, result in high workloads, creating a perfect storm. They note that

> *the irony, of course, is that these macro-level policy shifts inhibit the potential of a professionally curious approach because they result in practitioners having less time and fewer resources at their disposal … practitioners are being responsibilised to do something while simultaneously being denied the resources with which to do it.*
>
> (Phillips et al, 2024, p 333)

The authors point out that staff first need to be given the time to understand the root cause of people's problems (Phillips et al, 2024).

Increasing demand on services

More than half a million extra roles in social care will be needed over the next 15 years to keep up with demand, based on a growing older population and with vacancies in social care remaining around three times the national average of other sectors (Skills for Care, 2024). The impact of a reduced and reducing workforce is seen in high workloads. The second national SAR analysis (Preston-Shoot et al, 2024) identifies the impact of workloads (and the inferred restriction on practitioners' flexibility to use professional curiosity) in 61 (27 per cent) of the examined SAR reports, but this has not been translated into recommendations for system change. The authors observe that

> recommendations on workloads were noticeably missing, although one SAR did recommend that a system should be developed to cover worker absence. Another recommended that the local authority and NHS trust should develop an action plan to reduce resource pressures. Seeking assurance from health and social care operational and strategic managers that workloads are manageable and that supervision of cases involving adults at risk ensures that plans are implemented, and their outcomes reviewed.
>
> (Preston-Shoot et al, 2024, p 177)

As services have contracted, service delivery has become increasingly task-focused, rather than providing enough time to see the bigger picture. This squeezes the space in which professional curiosity can be encouraged, nurtured and developed.

Policy and legislative constraints

Identification of the need for greater professional curiosity in safeguarding adults practice in SARs and other reviews reflects the narrative in child protection and safeguarding practice first seen in the Munro Review (2010). In child protection practice, Dickens et al (2022) describe a 'subtle practice context' in which there are tensions between the wider societal and legal imperatives of respecting parents' rights and family privacy, building trusting relationships and acting to protect a child from abuse and harm. There are similar tensions for adult safeguarding practice, in which practitioners must navigate the policy, legal and values imperatives to respect autonomy and protect autonomy at the same time, while ensuring that those who are unable to protect themselves from abuse and neglect are supported to do so. Chapter 5 introduces you to some of the key legal and policy frameworks that guide practice, which would enable you to examine rights including some of the practice tensions. Policies and procedures should allow for professional discretion and flexibility. Engaging with policy-makers to advocate for more responsive frameworks would enable practitioners to exercise greater curiosity and judgement in their work.

Societal attitudes and stigma

Societal biases and stigma towards certain populations (eg people with mental health conditions, HIV/AIDS, physical disability, social housing tenants) can influence practitioners' attitudes and assumptions. This can lead to less curiosity and more judgemental practice, impacting the quality of care and investigation (Jackson-Best and Edwards, 2018).

Practitioners often face pressure to produce quick results, which can lead to superficial assessments and decision-making, undermining thorough investigative work. Media reporting on failures in a range of services – for example, within mental health (Precey, 2024) – often explains the failure of agencies to protect those in need or subject to abuse due to a 'lack of professional curiosity' by an individual practitioner. The appeal of this explanation is that it reduces the need for wider systematic questions and exploration of systemic issues.

Overarching political/cultural context

Burton and Revell (2018) argue that the political context in which organisations and the services they provide operate is inextricably linked to their culture, as it provides the backdrop to the changing social and political landscape, which filters down to individual practice encounters. They suggest that the complex interplay of the following factors constructs barriers to enacting professional curiosity:

- a contemporary society in which the vulnerable have become increasingly marginalised (and are frequently 'othered');
- market forces, increasingly driving risk-averse practices dominated by performance management indicators and paperwork, the 'proceduralisation' of social work practice (we would argue that includes other professional services, such as education, law enforcement and healthcare);
- leading to disconnection from frontline practice when the heart of practice is relational and emotional.

Conclusion

This chapter has explored some of the barriers to professional curiosity. Professional curiosity is essential for effective safeguarding adult practice, but it is often hindered by individual, organisational and systemic barriers. Organisational constraints, cultural and social norms, psychological factors and educational shortcomings all play a role in impeding curious behaviours. As mentioned in Chapter 1, a lack of professionally curious practice is often cited in SARs. A lot of SARs repeat phrases such as 'there were many examples in X's case where practitioners demonstrated a lack of professional curiosity'. Media reporting of tragic cases reinforces the public perception that individual practitioners are usually to blame, rather than asking questions about the wider system. Most professionals fully support the principle of professional curiosity, but a whole host of interrelated factors prevent them from consistently practising it in their day-to-day work.

Addressing these barriers requires a multifaceted approach, including enhanced training and development, fostering supportive organisational cultures, managing resource constraints and advocating for policy and systemic change. Creating an environment that supports and encourages professional curiosity can help social care practitioners to better understand and address the complex needs of their clients, ultimately leading to improved outcomes and well-being for the people that social care serves.

> ### KEY POINTS FROM THIS CHAPTER
>
> Potential barriers to professional curiosity include, but are not limited to:
>
> - personal issues (such as emotional exhaustion and burnout, compassion fatigue, secondary trauma, personal bias and assumptions, cognitive bias, lack of cultural curiosity, lack of confidence, fear of reaction, fear of making mistakes and professional deference);
> - case dynamics (such as limited knowledge, disguised compliance, the rule of optimism/minimising risk, normalisation and knowing but not knowing);
> - organisational issues (such as bureaucratic processes, inadequate supervision, resource constraints, increasing workload pressures, high workload and lack of time, organisational culture, insufficient training and development);
> - systemic factors (such as a climate of austerity, increasing demand for services, policy and legislative constraints, societal attitudes and stigma, overarching political/cultural context).

Further reading

Preston-Shoot, M, Braye, S, Doherty, C, Stacey, H, Hopkinson, P, Rees, K, Spreadbury, K and Taylor, G (2024) *Second National Analysis of Safeguarding Adult Reviews. Final report: Stage 2 Analysis – Analysis of Learning*. [online] Available at: https://tinyurl.com/48j2ar5v (accessed 13 November 2024).

Provides in depth analysis of learning from SARs.

3 Enablers of professional curiosity in safeguarding adult practice

CHAPTER OBJECTIVES

By end of this chapter, you should be able to:

- know what factors enable professional curiosity to flourish;
- identify strategies to help you pay better attention, increase your awareness and remain calm;
- challenge yourself to 'see more' by asking yourself 'What am I not seeing?';
- understand when your body is telling you something isn't right and how to use that 'gut feeling' to develop your curiosity;
- understand the importance of keeping the person central to all professional interventions;
- support yourself to have a learning mindset, even if that doesn't come naturally;
- understand and apply critical thinking and reflection to your interactions with adults.

Introduction

This chapter considers enablers of professional curiosity. It focuses on the individual and organisational factors that interact to produce conditions favourable to a curious, inquiring approach. The chapter discusses characteristics and attributes that foster professional curiosity and the ways you can take steps to become more self-aware and a curious practitioner through the lens of neuroscience. The role of organisations and managers in enabling curiosity is also considered.

Characteristics and attributes that foster curiosity practice

Kashdan et al (2018) highlight that naturally curious people seem to inherently possess skills including flexibility, the ability to adapt to changing situations, enjoyment of complex and abstract thinking, strong intellectual capacity and an ability to feel comfortable with uncertainty and anxiety. These attributes are key enablers of curiosity (Kashdan et al, 2018). Curiosity is not just a desirable quality but an essential skill for all involved in safeguarding adults (from healthcare workers to social workers, police officers, probation and the third sector). Frontline practitioners are placed in key positions that enable them to identify and raise concerns about abuse or neglect and intervene by taking action to support people to stay safe. Other attributes that enable curiosity to flourish include the ability to identify and manage risk and robust decision-making – including when working with agencies struggling to provide safe care in times of crises in recruitment and retention or when working with people whose intentions towards adults with care and support needs may not always be good/positive.

How to increase your own curiosity: insights from neuroscience

Our brains *predict* our reality (predictive processing)

Recent developments in neuroscience suggest that, rather than information we receive from our senses being the starting point of our experience, the brain tries to make predictions about the world based on our pre-existing '*mental models*' of the world (Clark, 2023, p xiii). Our brains try to make sense of our experience by making 'best guesses' about the causes of the sensory information received. Further information, as it becomes available (for example, as we look more closely), helps us to decide which prediction is correct. In this way, the brain tries to minimise errors. For example, if I see a black shape out of the corner of my eye, my brain predicts that I am seeing my black cat, who is usually around me. It is only when I look again in more detail that I notice that what I am actually seeing is a black coat on a chair. We frequently fill in gaps in our perceptions, creating the reality we *expect* to see, not what is really there. We can miss these prediction errors, and this leads to cognitive biases such as confirmation or optimism biases (Seth, 2021).

APPLYING CONCEPTS TO PRACTICE

Case study

Khalid, a social worker, and Beth, a housing officer, carried out a home visit to Mr Hunt after reports were received that he was neglecting his environment, which was now in a hazardous state. Khalid entered the property and was aware of a lot of

→

items in the environment, including piles of paper and boxes of books. Khalid was vaguely aware of a light fitting hanging from the ceiling. It was not until Beth drew his attention to it that Khalid realised what he'd thought was a light fitting was actually exposed wires coming from the ceiling, posing a significant risk of electrocution.

TASK

- What can we learn from predictive processing in this example?
- How might Khalid have expanded his field of awareness to notice the exposed wires?
- What else have you learnt from this example about the value of multidisciplinary working?

As a housing officer, Beth is more primed to see the dangers from exposed wires and identify them as a hazard because reviewing accommodation is part of her daily activity. Because Khalid *expected* to see a light fitting, his brain made a *prediction error* by filling in the gaps to create the reality he expected – that is, a hanging light fitting, rather than the exposed wires.

The impact of prior experiences

Clark (2023) discusses the impact of our prior experiences and prior beliefs on our brain's automatic predictions and warns about the dangers of unconscious bias. These are previous experiences we have had that shape the predictions or anticipations of what we will see in future experience. Relating this to the case study involving Khalid and Beth, Beth's prior experiences of working in the housing sector led her to anticipate potential issues with wiring in neglected properties. Khalid had less experience in this area so did not see the danger. Practitioners working with adults at risk of abuse or neglect must learn to look carefully to really *see* and be *fully aware* of the people and environments they visit. You must also be self-aware about your cultural beliefs and what has shaped these so you do not jump to wrong conclusions about what you see but instead use the relevant evidence base to inform your practice. Let's explore another case study and consider their implications for practice.

APPLYING CONCEPTS TO PRACTICE

Case study

Moira is a district nurse visiting Mr Dixon to monitor and manage his diabetes. Moira notices that Mr Dixon's wife seems very irritated with him, tutting and sighing as he tries to get his medication from its packaging to show the nurse. At one point,

> Mrs Dixon slaps her husband's hand out of the way and says, *'Oh for heaven's sake, let me do it or we'll be here all day.'*
>
> Moira remembers how frustrated her own mother used to be when Moira's grandmother needed to be cared for and thinks, *'No wonder the poor woman is annoyed.'*

TASK

- What can you learn from predictive processing in this scenario?
- How might Moira's prior experiences be impacting her approach in this scenario?
- How might Moira have interpreted this situation differently?
- How could you apply this learning to your own practice?

Moira has interpreted this incident in the context of her prior experience and felt sense when she connected her emotional response to her feelings when her mother was caring for her grandmother. As a consequence of the meaning she has made from the incident, Moira has normalised Mrs Dixon's behaviour and missed an opportunity to identify potential abuse and report it. Had the incident been reported to the local authority, action could have been taken to see Mr Dixon alone and engage him in a conversation about his wife's behaviour. Mrs Dixon may have been feeling stressed by her role as a carer and lost her temper, in which case the couple might benefit from additional support and advice. The incident could also be an indicator of long-standing domestic abuse within the marriage which would need to be carefully explored.

Thinking the unthinkable

Many people's prior experiences do not involve serious trauma or abuse. It can therefore be difficult to believe that crimes such as sexual abuse could be perpetrated against children, or adults with care and support needs (Malmedal, 2020). This is another type of confirmation bias, whereby evidence is sought to affirm a pre-held belief ('this couldn't possibly happen') and deny evidence that refutes it. You are encouraged to find ways to hold your prior experiences more lightly and keep your mind open to the possibility of abuse or neglect. Keeping an open mind and using evidence to inform practice enables effective curiosity.

For more examples and information on how our predictive brains can fill the gaps, see the YouTube video *Sine Wave Speech* (Moyle, 2014). You will find fragments of degraded speech that sound like white noise until you hear the sentence spoken in its entirety. After hearing the full sentence, the degraded sound can suddenly be heard clearly as our brain is now able to fill the gaps with the sound we expect to hear. A similar effect is found visually with Mooney images – again, these can be found online with an example described by Hutson (2023). On first viewing, the image seems to be a random set of black and white markings until you are told what to look for. With this cue, the brain is able to fill the gaps in the sensory information available and the picture emerges.

The role of emotion

Clarke (2023) suggests emotions are feelings constructed by our brains in response to the internal sensations in our bodies, which drive our decision-making about future actions. These are important in structuring your thoughts about the stories you hear, what you see and how you act when engaging with curiosity. Literature tells us that our bodily sensations (the way we feel within our bodies) have been shown to have an impact on which of our prior experiences we place more emphasis on, and which will influence our decision-making (Barrett, 2006, 2017). Indeed, Allen and Tsakiris (2018) describe the body as our 'first prior', to explain how we use the sensations we pick up from our bodies to inform our decision-making. Our past experience, combined with this 'felt sense', constructs emotions such as anxiety. Barrett (2021) describes how the sensation of a pounding heart could lead to different emotions being generated, depending on the circumstance. For example, awaiting test results could lead the brain to construct an emotion such as anxiety; at a fairground, it could construct excitement; and when exercising, the brain might construct the emotion of fatigue. The meaning our brain makes in each situation helps it to plan our next action and keep us safe. Our felt sense can literally affect what we see.

Why is this important in relation to professional curiosity?

Learning from predictive processing and constructed emotion shows that how we feel internally, and how we construct the world based on our prior experiences and anticipations, informs our behaviours and actions. Experiments with sine wave speech and Mooney images show that we fill the gaps where information is missing to try to make sense of the world around us. We only ever have a *partial view*: we can be sure that in every situation *we don't know more than we do know*. However, the brain is constantly making 'best guesses' about what is going to happen next based on sensory information received by the body and starts to act as if something is true – for example, that a trailing wire is a light fitting – thus making a significant difference to how we approach our interactions with the people with whom we work. Seth (2024) eloquently summarises current understanding of how the brain uses 'best guesses', which are often incorrect, the role of 'felt sense' and emotion in affecting our behaviour and the extent to which we can pick up our prediction errors. In the context of safeguarding adults work, this emphasises the importance of using curiosity to expand our field of awareness and see more of the world around us. Research tells us that how we use language and frame our prior experiences impacts how we view the world (Clark, 2023).

APPLYING CONCEPTS TO PRACTICE
The importance of framing

Look at the following three statements and think about the impact of how they have been framed.

Statement 1

Mental health hospitals are full of people with complex conditions that lead to agitated behaviour. It is unavoidable that there will be physical incidents arising between the patients and it seems disproportionate to raise them all as safeguarding concerns.

Statement 2

There has been under-reporting of safeguarding concerns in mental health hospitals where people with care and support needs arising from their mental health issues have been assaulted by other patients.

Statement 3

I feel afraid to come out of my room in the hospital as there is a man who pushed me against the wall last week. I know he's very unwell, but he is bigger than me and the last time it really hurt my shoulder. I'm worried that if he did it again, I might be seriously hurt. I haven't been able to talk to anyone about my worries, so I just stay in my room.

These statements are all related to incidents of assault in mental health hospitals. The way they are framed significantly impacts how much importance we would place on raising a safeguarding concern when there has been an assault by one patient against another in the hospital. If we can inquire into the nature and origin of our beliefs and develop a better understanding of how and why they arose, we are able to loosen our hold on them and become better able to consider and be open to alternatives (Zhu et al, 2021). For example, in the case of Moira and Mr Dixon (discussed earlier in this chapter), Moira's attention was placed on the prior experience of her mother caring for her grandmother, which affected how she interpreted the slap by Mrs Dixon. It highlights the importance of being open-minded and self-aware, and of using critical reflection and analysis to inform your practice. This increases the likelihood of curiosity as it increases the potential for reframing of your prior experience. In the case of Moira, working through and inquiring into her beliefs about her mother's experience of caring for her grandmother could help her to question her interpretation of those events and relax her hold on them. This would enable her to see an incident of abuse by a carer towards the cared-for person. Critical reflection and analysis are key facilitators of professional curiosity. We shape our reality based on our anticipations, picking up prediction errors and learning from them to modify what we see and how we interpret our experience. Our ability to successfully pick up errors and see more of what is really there is affected by several factors, including:

- stress and pressure;
- mood or emotional state;
- our internal state, for example, whether we are hungry, thirsty, cold, tired or have consumed caffeine or other chemical substances;
- which of our prior experiences we pay more attention to or place more emphasis on;
- our flexibility and ability to hold our beliefs and prior experiences with less rigidity;
- the way a situation has been framed (in the case of Moira and Mr Dixon, Moira had framed Mr Dixon as a source of annoyance and frustration and Mrs Dixon as a victim having to suffer the irritation) and our capacity to reframe it;
- how quickly we are trying to perceive something from another perspective.

The impact of stress and pressure

When our bodies are either physically or mentally stressed, our nervous system responds by preparing our bodies for 'fight or flight'. The physical effects of the stress response include increased heart rate, rapid breathing, dilated pupils, muscle tension, sweating, increased blood pressure, reduced digestive activity and dulled pain reception (Harvard Health Publishing, 2020). While these effects may have been helpful when we needed to run from or fight a predator, they are unhelpful in situations that call for curiosity. This is because stress narrows our focus onto the perceived stress factor, which can limit our awareness of peripheral details and make it challenging to see the bigger picture. Stress also impairs concentration and our ability to maintain attention – which, as described above, limits how much of a situation you can really 'see'. Stress can also cause cognitive overload, making it difficult to process information effectively and it impairs problem-solving and leads to more rigid thought processes, limiting your awareness of alternative solutions (Córdova et al, 2023).

Practices that support curiosity

Many people are unaware of their inner felt sense most of the time and struggle to report how their body feels. Barrett (2006, 2017, 2021) notes that there is a deep connection between our present perceptions and past experiences, and that our brains tend to assign more importance to predictions associated with strong emotions, making us susceptible to confirmation and other types of bias. Stress can alter our emotional state and influence the weight we give to our predictions. Heightening our awareness of our bodily sensations can enhance our ability to understand how emotions influence the importance we assign to our predictions. Thus, by being aware of how we feel internally, we are more likely to recognise that there could be another way to perceive a situation (Moira might be able to see she had recognised Mrs Dixon's behaviour as a natural response to frustration, rather than as an assault on an adult with care and support needs). Kahneman (2011) notes that to access more of our awareness, we need to *slow down* our thinking. This supports us to work through our assumptions and beliefs, improve our attention and capacity to pick up prediction errors, and take time to work through how our prior experiences could be impacting our thoughts, feelings and bodily sensations.

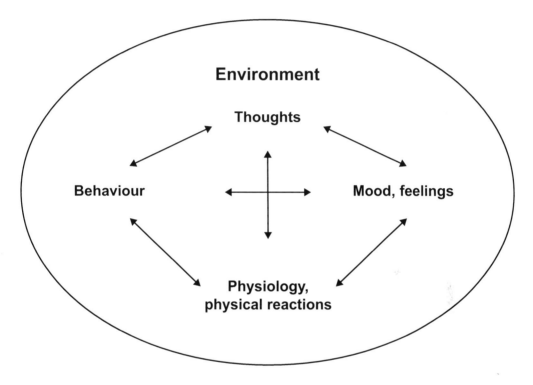

Figure 3.1 Adapted from Padesky and Mooney (1990)

TASK

Think about an encounter you have had – perhaps something you experienced as stressful or difficult – and list your:

- bodily sensations;
- thoughts;

- feelings/emotions;
- behaviour.

Can you identify any patterns? How did your bodily sensations affect your response in the situation? How might this situation have been different if you had been able to slow down your thinking/notice your felt sense and emotions in the moment?

This exercise helps us to get in touch with how our felt senses might be influencing our thoughts, feelings and behaviours. It helps to put us back in touch with our bodies so we can 'listen' to our 'gut feelings' to help us articulate what is concerning us and start to seek evidence to support or refute our concerns.

APPLYING CONCEPTS TO PRACTICE

Case study

Adaku is a 32 year-old Nigerian social worker who has worked in the United Kingdom for seven years. She has been asked to carry out a review for Joe, who lives in a residential care setting for people with learning difficulties. Joe has been putting on weight and concerns have been expressed by the speech and language therapist (SALT) that the provider is not adhering to Joe's care plan by failing to provide him with opportunities for exercise and failing to support a healthy diet. Adaku's first instinct is to advise her manager that Joe's annual review will take place in a couple of months and these issues could be picked up then by a member of the reviewing team.

When she pauses to reflect, Adaku realises that she is experiencing discomfort in her body when she thinks about this review and recognises that she has been trying to avoid doing it. With this knowledge, Adaku thinks about why she might be avoiding doing the review. She identifies that the provider manager, an older, white, British male, reminds her of her first manager when she came to work in the United Kingdom. Adaku had felt undermined by her manager and the memories of that time are linked with feelings of powerlessness and oppression. She feels that the provider manager doesn't listen to or respect her, and she realises she is feeling anxiety about potentially having to challenge him about Joe's care plan.

As part of her planning for the visit, Adaku decides to invite the SALT to be part of the review meeting as the SALT will be able to go through her concerns and put forward the evidence to show that Joe's care plan is not being met adequately. Adaku also decides to cover the topic of weight management as the first item on the agenda to ensure it is covered as she has experienced the manager trying to deflect concerns by talking about aspects of the care plan that are going well.

Adaku carries out a short attention practice before the meeting to slow her thinking and support her body to stay calm. During the meeting, the manager attempts to

> talk about Joe's friendship with another resident when Adaku tries to address weight management. Having anticipated this, Adaku politely states that it's good to hear Joe has made a friend but that there is a need to discuss his diet and exercise first.
>
> A plan is made at the meeting to support Joe to have a healthier diet and it is agreed that he will be taken swimming twice a week. Adaku sets a date for the first swimming session to have been completed and writes this into the care plan. She makes another date to carry out a follow-up review and makes it clear that she expects the actions from the care plan will have started by then. After the meeting, the SALT asks what will happen if the swimming hasn't been arranged by the next review. Adaku says she will phone to check progress and restate the importance of the swimming so if it has not been set up by the next meeting without good reason, she will talk to her manager about notifying the commissioning team as the provider organisation will not be fulfilling its contractual arrangements.

Self-care

In a culture of stress and pressure, where waiting lists abound and there is an ever-increasing strain in the health, social care, policing and third sector systems, many practitioners believe they are too busy to make time for mindfulness, counselling, coaching or other well-being activities. However, we argue that the stressful cultures in which we work make engagement in some of these activities vital, particularly for those to whom curiosity does not come naturally. Research evidence suggests that giving active attention to the influence of our embodied mind, our prior experiences and the impact of thinking too quickly can support us to develop our curiosity to function in modern safeguarding practice. The good news is that even as little as one minute a day engaging in a mindfulness activity has benefits, as our capacity to build our attention is strengthened over time (Gibson, 2019). Could you give some time – however small – to any of these activities to enhance your curiosity and practice?

REFLECTIVE QUESTIONS

- What is stopping you from being more curious?
- What is preventing you from carrying out some kind of mindfulness activity each day?
- How can you remove obstacles to carrying out some kind of mindfulness activity each day? How could your manager support you to do this?
- How much time could you commit to using mindfulness techniques each day? One minute? Five minutes? Ten minutes? More?
- How could you build this activity into your daily routine?

APPLYING CONCEPTS TO PRACTICE
Case study

Ewa is a crisis case manager in a mental health service and has been asked to carry out an urgent visit to Velma Weber, a 27 year-old woman who is reported to be extremely low in mood – possibly suicidal. The call came in late on a dark, wet November day and Ewa is tired and cold when she arrives at Velma's property in a deprived area of the city. There are several people shouting in the otherwise quiet street when Ewa arrives and parks her car. One of the people approaches as she gets out of the car and asks if she's got a light for cigarette. Ewa feels intimidated, says 'no, sorry' and hurries to Velma's flat. She knocks on the door, which is opened a crack, and Velma peers round asking, 'Who is it?' Ewa introduces herself and shows her ID badge. She asks if she can come in, but Velma says it's not a good time as she's making something to eat. Ewa can hear what sounds like a large dog barking in the house and the sound echoes around. Ewa feels a strong urge to leave the property as she feels unsafe. Ewa accepts that Velma is busy and doesn't want a visit now and rushes back to her car. As she locks the car door and puts the heating on, she feels a rush of relief through her body.

TASK

- How is Ewa's 'felt sense' impacting on her actions in this scenario?
- How might Ewa's prior experiences be impacting her approach?
- How might Ewa have managed this situation differently but still remained safe?
- How could you apply this learning to your own practice?

Holding difficult conversations and challenging

Some individuals, families or providers can become very skilled at diverting a conversation away from the topic the professional wants to discuss. Nicolas (2016) points out that this can result in the focus shifting away from the subject of the safeguarding enquiry or complex assessment.

Tips to support you to hold difficult conversations

- Plan in advance to ensure there will be time to cover the essential elements of the conversation.
- Think about any particular issues that could arise. Do you have any prior experiences that relate to the person or situation you are dealing with that may be

impacting your body sensations, feelings, thoughts or behaviours? What can you do to minimise their impact?

- Take some time before the meeting to carry out a body scan or short mindfulness practice to help slow down your thinking and reactions and stay calm.
- Keep the agenda focused on the topics you need to cover. Be clear and unambiguous, and return consistently to the point that needs to be discussed, regardless of diversion tactics used.
- Have the courage to address the difficult topic and don't find reasons to avoid it. Focus on the needs of the person.
- Be non-confrontational and non-blaming – stick to the facts.
- Remember that your primary responsibility is to the person you are supporting, not the family/provider.
- Have evidence to back up what you say. Ensure decision-making is justifiable and transparent.
- Show empathy, consideration and compassion; be real and honest.
- Demonstrate congruence, making sure your tone, body language and content of speech are consistent.
- Acknowledge 'gut feelings', sharing these with other professionals and seeking evidence to support or refute those intuitions.
- Understand the elements and indicators of behavioural change.
- Carry a healthy scepticism.
- Understand the complexities of disguised compliance.

Never be concerned about asking an obvious question and share concerns with colleagues and managers. A 'fresh pair of eyes' looking at a case can help practitioners and organisations to maintain a clear focus on good practice and risk assessment and develop a critical mindset.

Robust information gathering

The importance of carefully checking the history of a case was discussed in Chapter 2. Doing this will highlight important information such as previous safeguarding concerns, alert practitioners to known risks and help to identify what the person does and doesn't want (including during a crisis). Reading and familiarising yourselves with the case history also enables you to identify any individuals in the person's network who may be known not to operate in the person's best interests. It will also help you to identify actions that have already been taken and other professionals who have been or currently are involved. Knowledge of these aspects will inform next steps and actions. If a case is to be passed to another practitioner, a detailed and comprehensive handover should be provided to familiarise the new worker with the case and the current risk(s) and plans already implemented. It takes time to go through a case record, particularly if there is a long history of involvement, but not doing so could mean failing to take important information into consideration. It is important to set aside time in advance to read records and familiarise yourself with the case history. It is also important to ask key questions as you acquaint yourself with the case history. An analytical practitioner takes an approach that repeatedly questions the information available, and actively considers different interpretations of the same information. It is also important to have a critical mindset, to help you to question whether there is anything odd or unexpected about information received or experience observed in order to know when more information or evidence might be needed. Chatfield (2018) points out that we should not accept information at face value. Scepticism and objectivity are required to establish whether information is correct and can be trusted (Laming, 2003). Taking such approaches can help you to guard against the risks from biased information (information that is one-sided and creates a distorted account of the way things are), or information acting to support your own confirmation bias. As discussed in earlier chapters, cognitive biases are known to adversely affect outcomes across human professions in medicine (Croskerry, 2013), policing (Afful, 2018), social work (Featherston et al, 2019) and nursing (Martin et al, 2022). Cognitive biases occur when we take mental 'short-cuts', form judgements and make predictions in the absence of certainty or having the full information. When this happens, our brains fill the gaps with predictions based on prior experiences and these can sometimes be incorrect (prediction errors). For a more extensive discussion of the many types of cognitive bias, see Korteling and Toet (2020). Interrogating the cogency, reliability or accuracy of the information or evidence can therefore help us to assess the degree of weight we should attribute to the information.

Questions to help establish the cogency, reliability or accuracy of information

- Who and where did the information/evidence come from?
- Why was the information/evidence given?
- How reliable is the source of the information/evidence?
- Do I believe the information/evidence?
- If I don't believe it, what might be the hidden intentions behind the information/evidence?
- Do I have proof that the information/evidence is correct?
- Can I verify/check the accuracy of the information/evidence using a reliable source to check what is really going on?
- Once I have done this, what action can I take?

APPLYING CONCEPTS TO PRACTICE
Case study

You have received a safeguarding concern from the son of one of the adults with whom you work. The son says his sister, who manages his mother's finances, is using her money to fund a holiday and a new car for her own son.

TASK

- Use the questions (listed above), to help you to establish the cogency, reliability or accuracy of information. Below are some example answers for you to refer to.

Who and where did the information/evidence come from?

From the adult's son.

Why was the information/evidence given?

Because the son alleges his sister is using his mother's finances inappropriately and there is possible financial abuse.

How reliable is the source of the information/evidence?

You may already know the dynamics in this family; there may be previous safeguarding enquiries on the adult's record. You will need to check the history of the case to gain some perspective on how reliable this information might be. Is there a history of family conflict? Has the adult expressed her wishes about who should manage her finances? Have concerns of this nature been received before and what was the outcome?

Do I believe the information/evidence?

We should seriously consider all safeguarding concerns raised, but we may still start to form a view about whether, based on the information gathered to date, we believe the information. Be sure to guard against confirmation bias; just because this issue hasn't been reported before doesn't mean it can't happen.

If I don't believe it, what might be the hidden intentions behind the information/evidence?

Does the son want to take on the management of his mother's finances? What might be his motive for this? Is there conflict in the family? Is he seeking financial gain?

Do I have proof that the information/evidence is correct?

Consider whether you already have enough information to take a view on this.

→

Can I verify/check the accuracy of the information/evidence using a reliable source to check what is really going on?

Do you know whether the adult has mental capacity? Would you be able to speak to her directly about this? Are there multi-agency partners who may have information to support or refute this allegation? Is there a Lasting Power of Attorney (for finance and property) in place?

Once I have done this, what action can I take?

If you remain uncertain about whether abuse or neglect has occurred or whether there is a risk of abuse or neglect of an adult with care and support needs who is not able to protect themselves, you must raise an enquiry for further enquiries to be made.

Curious organisations

Research and analysis of SARs have highlighted that a culture of curiosity must be owned by individuals (frontline practitioners), management and organisation for curiosity to thrive (Dickens et al 2023; Kedge and Appleby, 2009; Preston-Shoot et al, 2024; Thacker et al, 2020).

APPLYING CONCEPT TO PRACTICE

Safeguarding Adult Review: Issy

Lacy et al (2021) carried out a SAR concerning Issy, a 26 year-old woman with congenital myopathy. Issy died from a heart attack following sepsis because of infected pressure ulcers. She experienced complex cardiac and respiratory problems, pain and severe mobility issues, becoming increasingly socially isolated. Practitioners working with Issy *'saw but did not "see" the awfulness of her situation'*. It is reported that many people were desensitised to the level of neglect she experienced from being left in a smelly, soiled bed, unable to move. The authors of the SAR report attribute this phenomenon to a type of cognitive bias that they describe as tunnel vision, *'working to maintain a task focus in pressured work environments which increases the risk of staff inadvertently becoming desensitised to and dehumanising people'* (Lacy et al, 2021, p 3).

In a pressured situation, we can spotlight our focus to the immediate task which makes things appear more manageable but without the 'bird's eye view' that enables us to see the bigger picture. Practitioners may also have experienced 'groupthink', a type of cognitive bias where people set aside their own beliefs or doubts to conform with the perceived opinion of the rest of the group.

TASK

- What can we learn from predictive processing and neuroscience in relation to the internal feelings, thoughts, emotions and behaviours of practitioners working with Issy?
- How might practitioners have increased their ability to 'see' the full extent of Issy's situation?
- How might practitioners have reduced the impact of their cognitive biases through reflection on action?
- What reflective questions could practitioners have asked themselves to increase the extent to which they could 'see' Issy's situation?
- How could managers support their practitioners to be more curious about Issy's situation?

The role of managers

The role of managers and organisations in creating a culture of curiosity is explored in depth by Thacker et al (2020) and in analysis of child protection practice reviews of serious cases in England by Dickens et al (2023). Chapters 2 and 5 identify that the role of line managers and organisations is crucially important in supporting frontline practitioners and a key facilitator of professional curiosity. Thacker et al (2020) notes that the practice frameworks adopted by agencies, their learning and development, offers to support understanding, skilful use of legislation and a willingness to work with other organisations all contribute to the development of a curious culture.

Enablers of curiosity include using reflection and critical analysis in supervision processes, team meetings, quality assurance systems and, importantly, modelling of such an approach throughout the organisation – particularly by managers and leaders. Good leadership skills include commitments to lifelong learning and development, use of evidence-based practice, effective workload management, adequate resources and support, effective commissioning and compassion/kindness. A good organisation listens to and co-creates delivery of resources and interventions that support the needs and outcomes of its employees. It involves employees in evaluating what works and gaps in resources, including learning and development. In addition, a good organisation involves people who use services in exploring what works when commissioning services.

Research evidence demonstrates that organisational culture shapes conditions for continuing professional development and assists practitioners to keep their learning up to date (Mlambo et al, 2021). Organisations can support development of curiosity in the workforce by providing sufficient training and learning opportunities to pique the interest of their staff. Delivering training in ways that stimulate and engage learners is essential for supporting the development of curiosity (Thacker et al, 2020).

Organisations and line managers are encouraged to use practice approaches that build relationships of trust with people and communities (including frontline practitioners). The practice framework set by the leadership, and expectations around how it operates, are significant. For example, the strengths-based models of practice put conversations between equals at the heart of practice, focusing on the strengths in the person's life, working with them to identify the outcomes they want to achieve and enabling practitioners, line managers and organisations to learn. Key questions are:

- What is important to the person (employees, people who use services and their families)?
- What are their strengths and talents?
- What is working well and what do they want to change?
- What would they like to achieve?
- How would they like to be supported?

For more reading on models of practice for strategic leaders and managers in developing and modelling professional curiosity, see Thacker et al (2020).

Enablers of professional curiosity: a case example

The case study below presents an alternative version of events arising from the same scenario presented in the previous chapter, but where measures have been taken to enhance curiosity and curious practice.

APPLYING CONCEPTS TO PRACTICE

Case study

Social worker Jo has been allocated the case of Pat following a referral from the GP, who has reported that Pat isn't coping at home. Jo puts some time into her busy calendar to read Pat's record carefully. She learns that there have been several safeguarding concerns raised previously about financial abuse by Pat's son, who has now moved out of Pat's home. There is a risk recorded on Pat's record as her son has a history of aggression towards professionals and that it is not advisable to visit alone. She can see that there have been long-standing concerns about self-neglect.

Reading records and collating a good case history is a vital to alert professionals to the current and accumulating or escalating risks.

Jo rings the GP to gather more information and suggests they do a joint visit so the GP can check Pat's health. Jo also mentions that Pat has a son who has been aggressive in the past. He is not supposed to be there but it's not advisable to visit alone.

Working in partnership with other professionals increases curiosity, as it introduces, respects and values new perspectives and different expertise, and brings an opportunity to reflect.

After parking her car, Jo carries out a short body scan to slow down her thought processes, improve her ability to pay attention and reduce the impact of strong emotion on her decision-making.

Jo knocks confidently on the door, which is opened by a man in a suit who seems irritated and flustered; Jo thinks he must be Pat's son. The GP advises they have come to visit Pat to do some health and well-being checks. Pat's son, Martin, doesn't look pleased but allows them inside. Jo and the GP exchange a concerned look. The GP indicates that she will see Pat alone to examine her.

If there are safeguarding concerns, it is important to *find a way for a professional to see the person alone* so they can speak freely.

Jo and the GP squeeze past large numbers of hoarded possessions to Pat's bedroom, which smells strongly of urine. The GP introduces herself and Jo to Pat. Jo takes Martin through to the kitchen saying she would like to talk to him about how he's getting on looking after his mum. Martin tries to divert Jo by complaining about social workers interfering. Jo remembers a course she did on 'managing difficult conversations assertively' and politely steers back to her agenda by saying she understands but they have a responsibility to make sure Pat gets the health and care she needs.

Good-quality training equips professionals to spot the signs of possible abuse and identify when to dig deeper.

Martin says he's only staying a couple of days and he'll be getting his own place soon. He says his mum is very demanding, and it really gets on his nerves. Jo asks whether he's ever lost his temper with Pat. 'No, of course not,' he replies.

Being a curious practitioner, Jo *doesn't take this at face value* and decides to seek more evidence about Pat's relationship with her son. She is mindful of the safeguarding concerns on Pat's record.

Meanwhile, the GP talks to Pat about how things are at home. She asks whether Pat feels safe at home. Pat looks worried. She says her son is a good boy but can have a temper. The GP asks if he's ever hurt Pat. Pat says, 'Well all men can be a bit rough, can't they.' The GP asks Pat to describe what she means by this. Pat says he can be 'a bit grabby'.

The GP has used 'routine enquiry' – the process of asking questions to allow a person to disclose domestic abuse on all contacts with professionals. The GP keeps Pat at the heart of the discussion about safeguarding concerns.

Martin and Jo return to the room. The GP says she is very worried about Pat's health and thinks it would be advisable that she come to the surgery for more tests today. She says she will arrange transport. As Jo goes to say goodbye to Pat, she notices bruises on Pat's arm.

Once outside, the GP and Jo share their concerns about the bruising, Pat's disclosure and Martin's frustration. They think they have enough evidence to raise a safeguarding concern. An urgent safeguarding discussion takes place, which includes the police.

A plan is put in place to bring Pat to the surgery that afternoon and Jo arranges a respite placement to be on standby. At the surgery, Pat discloses physical violence by her son and an examination reveals her body is covered in bruises. Pat says she wants to live at home but wants her son to live somewhere else. She wants him to be less stressed so he won't hurt her. Pat moves to temporary respite care until she can safely return home.

Reflective questions to support practitioners working with adults

Britten and Whitby (2018), in their book *Self-Neglect: Learning from Life*, and HM Inspectorate of Probation (2022) offer different practice frameworks to inform practice. Writing from the context of children and families social work, Broadhurst et al (2010) advise that regular reflection is likely to lead to better critical analytical skills. The authors compiled a series of reflective questions that practitioners can ask themselves and managers can ask practitioners, which can be applied to safeguarding adult practice. These questions are designed to stimulate curiosity and prompt reflection on whether practitioners have done all they can to safeguard the adult with whom they are working.

- Am I curious about what I am seeing and learning in my work with this person?
- What am I not seeing?
- If I have a 'gut feeling' about this situation, why is that? What is my body telling me? What is concerning me and how can I find evidence to support my gut feeling?
- Am I keeping the person at the centre of my work with them?
- Have I prioritised the safety of the person?
- Have I taken account of the person's strengths in their situation?
- Did I involve the person fully in making decisions? What more could I have done?
- Do I know the person's view of their situation, needs or risks? If not, how can I establish their view?

- Have I done all I can to facilitate the person's involvement in my work with them – for example, by addressing any communication or language issues?
- Am I receptive to new information, even if it challenges my pre-existing beliefs about the case? Would I be prepared to change my theory if new information challenged it?
- Have I thoroughly read the case history and cross-referenced with other records where necessary?
- How can I find out more information about the background to this case?
- Have I shared information with those who need to know?
- If I feel stressed or overwhelmed, what can I do to get support?
- If I have felt intimidated or anxious about the case, what support can I seek? Has this affected my judgement?
- Am I using supervision to reflect on my cases to understand what is happening, rather than just to discuss workload?
- Have I assessed the mental capacity of the adult and documented my findings?
- Have I considered executive/functional, as well as decisional mental capacity?
- Have I carried out an assessment of risk and documented my findings?
- Have I considered whether the adult may be being coerced or controlled?
- Have I called a multidisciplinary meeting if I am feeling stuck with this case?
- Am I genuinely committed to ongoing learning and development? When was the last entry on my CPD log?
- Do I have any knowledge or skills gaps regarding my casework?

Conclusion

This chapter has been focused on enablers of professional curiosity, how you can increase your own curiosity and how managers and organisations can support you to do that. It drew from neuroscience and examined the impact of not seeing reality as it is, the implications for practice for misinterpreting situations involving the people with whom we work and why it is important to be self-aware about these. It offered suggestions and techniques to support you to see more, listen to your bodies and understand the impact of your prior experiences to address potential cognitive biases. The chapter encourages you to take responsibility for your own mental well-being and keep up to date with your learning and development. It also encourages organisations and line managers to create a culture where curiosity is enabled. Most of all, it encourages practitioners and organisations and systems to foster a culture of practice where the well-being of the person at the centre of safeguarding enquiries becomes central to all activity, so their concerns, wishes and the things that are important to them are truly heard.

KEY POINTS FROM THIS CHAPTER

You can promote professional curiosity by:

- reading the case history to familiarise yourself with the person at the centre of safeguarding enquiry before a visit;
- slowing down and remaining calm; take a minute before a visit, meeting, or encounter to clear your mind, calm your body's fight/flight responses and focus on your breathing;
- taking a minute after the event to ask yourself 'What is my body telling me?', 'What am I not seeing?', 'What did I miss?', 'What should I have asked?' 'What do I need to do next?';
- using practice frameworks to support decision-making;
- grounding your decisions in evidence;
- using critical reflection and analysis;
- providing training to enable practitioners to keep up to date with the knowledge and skills required for effective safeguarding practice.

Further reading

Clark, A (2023) *The Experience Machine.* Harmondsworth: Penguin.

Provides insight into how our past experiences shape our predictions and future experiences. This book will help you to examine your own biases, what has shaped these and their potential implications for practice.

Seth, A (2024) Consciousness in Humans and in Other Things. [online] Available at: https://tinyurl.com/m6hmvm6m (accessed 13 November 2024).

Essential reading with an eloquent summary of how the brain uses 'best guesses' which are often incorrect including the role of 'felt sense' and emotion on our behaviour.

Thacker, H Anka, A and Penhale, B (2020) *Professional Curiosity in Safeguarding Adults: Strategic Briefing.* Dartington: Research in Practice.

Examine the barriers and facilitators of professional curiosity and partnership work in safeguarding adults. Draws from analysis of SARs.

4 Application of professional curiosity to practice

CHAPTER OBJECTIVES

By the end of this chapter, you should be able to:

- understand more about the skills, attributes and values required for applying professional curiosity in safeguarding adults work;
- apply professional curiosity to practice in a multi-agency context;
- recognise the consequences of not using curiosity in safeguarding practice;
- understand what best practice looks like based on examples from SARs, CSPR and other scenarios;
- reflect on situations you have experienced, observed or heard about in this context.

Introduction

As the previous chapters have covered, professional curiosity needs to be a central feature when working with adults who may be at risk of, or experiencing, harm or abuse. In Chapter 1, Table 1.1 set out a summary of the core skills, abilities and attributes required for engaging in professional curiosity practice in work done with those owed a duty of care and protection from abuse, neglect and harm and their families and carers. This chapter will look at some of those in more depth. The chapter looks at examples from reviews that have taken place when a child or adult has died or come to serious harm to see where, and more importantly why, some of the barriers and enablers discussed in Chapters 2 and 3 had a significant impact. Throughout, you are encouraged to consider the concept of professional curiosity in a multi-agency context – what it means to a wide range of people, including people with lived experience (PWLE) and organisations.

Unpacking the concept of professional curiosity

The role of SABs includes direct support of local safeguarding adults' partnerships, and a large part of its work includes finding ways to translate many safeguarding or social care concepts such as professional curiosity to support effective communication and understanding between agencies when they work together. Discussions in a number of local safeguarding forums have made it clear that these concepts (eg professional curiosity) can sometimes feel 'professionalised', which in practice risks excluding those who would not identify themselves as such or indeed to the false belief that someone else – a professional – is the only one who can do something or hold responsibility for something. Using these phrases is a useful shorthand to explain a concept, but this only works if all parties involved know and understand the concept. The biggest danger of this perception in practice is that something doesn't happen – 'it's not my job/role'; there might be an action missed or information that doesn't get shared. A different way to think may be not as 'the curiosity of a professional' but rather the curiosity that is sanctioned because of your working role – permission to be 'nosy', to ask questions that might be seen as probing. In our multi-agency safeguarding partnerships, the concept of professional curiosity is often translated as 'being interested' – a very basic term, but a useful springboard that allows for more in-depth discussion and exploration with colleagues who are often in a position to see things that happen or ask questions, but may not initially feel it is their core role.

Safeguarding Adults Reviews (SARs – for adults), Child Safeguarding Practice Reviews (CSPRs) and analysis of Domestic Abuse Related Death Reviews (DARDRs) (for adults but children may be involved) all take place for one main reason: to look back in more detail at a situation where a child or adult has died or come to serious harm, and to identify where something could have been done differently. This is vital for us, as professionals, agencies and others involved, to learn relevant lessons and prevent that harm from happening again wherever possible. It is all about how the agencies involved can work more effectively together by identifying those opportunities for best practice. Several themes are common to all these types of reviews, and one is a lack of professional curiosity, as mentioned in earlier chapters. When searching the National SARs library, more than 650 SAR documents since 2019 have referenced a lack of professional curiosity as an issue in the case under review. In safeguarding children practice, a published summary of Serious Case Reviews that took place between 1988 and 2019 (before a move to local Child Safeguarding Practice Reviews and rapid reviews) noted that *'the 2005–07 review was the first of the overview reports to use the phrase 'professional curiosity', however similar ideas appeared in the previous overviews'* (Department for Education, 2022, p 6). The SCRs identified that

> *parental accounts and the views of other professionals were often not sufficiently questioned or challenged; striking a balance between observing and questioning safeguarding and child protection concerns and building effective relationships with families can be difficult; practitioners need training and supervision to think compassionately and not get stuck in 'rigid thinking'.*
>
> (Department for Education, 2022, p 7)

As mentioned in Chapter 2, the second national SAR analysis, completed between 2019 and 2023, mentioned the absence of professional curiosity. This was a feature in 44 per cent of the reviews (Preston-Shoot et al, 2024).

Safeguarding adults is everybody's business, so concepts like professional curiosity need to be embedded within a strong multi-agency context, no matter what the working role (and that includes unpaid roles, volunteers, informal carers, etc). Like many skills, it is the application in practice that makes the difference, and that starts with listening, having a clear understanding, support in developing and confidence in using professional curiosity. Table 4.1 provides four types of listeners identified by Hargie (2016, p 192), this provides fascinating insights into how we listen.

Table 4.1 Four types of listeners

People-oriented listeners	Primary concern is for others' feelings and needs. Can be distracted away from the task owing to this focus on psycho-emotional perspectives. We seek them out when we need a listening ear. They are good helpers.
Task-oriented listeners	Mainly concerned with getting the business done. Do not like discussing what they see as irrelevant information or having to listen to 'long-winded' people. Can be insensitive to the emotional needs of others.
Content-oriented listeners	These are analytical people who enjoy dissecting information and carefully scrutinising it. They often focus on the literal meaning of what has been said. They want to hear all sides and leave no stone unturned, however long the process. They can be slow to make decisions as they are never quite sure that they have garnered all the necessary information. Are good mediators.
Time-oriented listeners	Their main focus is upon getting tasks completed within set timeframes. They see time as a valuable commodity, not to be wasted. They are impatient with what they see as 'prevaricators' and can be prone to jump to conclusions before they have heard all the information.

Taken from: Hargie (2016, p 192).

REFLECTIVE QUESTIONS

- Take some time to reflect on the different types of listeners presented in Table 4.1.
- What type of listener are you and what are the implications for using professional curiosity practice in safeguarding work?

Applying time and workload pressures to any service or individual can narrow practice focus to simply the function you are there to carry out, which can reduce professional curiosity (Thacker et al, 2020). Too often, this also diminishes the person themselves and reduces them solely to the problem you are there to 'fix'. This is as true in safeguarding as any other context, with the sole aim being to 'make the person safe'. Being safe is a subjective, existential and complex concept. Living is not without risk, and people think about risk in different ways. So, to know what being safe means to an individual, ensuring their voice is integral to any process or intervention, means seeking understanding of their unique experience and the context to any safeguarding risk or concern, using your professional curiosity.

The heart of listening

Listening is central to safeguarding work and professional curiosity. Listening involves the ability to attend to, remember, understand and respond to others. Listening includes affirming the individual's right to be heard and involves both verbal and non-verbal communication. These are central to rapport-building and a relationship of trust. Weinstein et al (2022) identify three key qualities shown by a listener in high-quality listening as giving undivided attention, showing understanding, and positive intention. High-quality listening includes showing genuine interest, care and curiosity. We can demonstrate these attributes by not interrupting the speaker when they are speaking, including not checking our mobile phone while they are speaking. We can also show understanding by nodding, paraphrasing or clarifying. Likewise, we show genuine interest, care and curiosity by being non-judgemental and providing validation. High-quality listening is also associated with providing both social and psychological support. Weinstein et al (2022) point out that high-quality listening is impactful when working with deeply personal or threatening disclosures.

Safeguarding incidents can often be distressing for the adult involved, and for those around them. While some adults may be fully aware of what is happening to them, due to their needs they may be unable to protect themselves from harm. That loss of control can be compounded where professionals or organisations 'take over' without meaningful discussion or offering choice to the person, creating additional dependency, limiting the adult's own agency. From the beginning to the end of a safeguarding enquiry, the adult or their advocate should be actively involved and listened to. This is more than just about asking what they want at the beginning (although very important), but also:

- keeping them updated on any progress;
- helping them to be part of the process where relevant;
- supporting and empowering them to shape outcomes where possible.

A good example of the difference this might make is reflected in the Oldham SAR of Derek (Berry, 2022), which followed on from a Learning from Lives and Deaths Review (LeDeR), carried out for anyone with a learning disability or autism). Derek was 69 when he died due to diabetic complications. He was found dead in his own home on 6 December 2019. He had a diagnosed learning disability and other health conditions, including diabetes. Derek was known to a range of services relating to his medical, housing and social needs, with concerns about possible self-neglect and about how he managed his diabetes. The review included comments from Derek's niece about his perception of his situation and how agencies worked with him:

Application of professional curiosity to practice • 69

- His physical health significantly deteriorated and his mobility was reduced.
- He did not feel safe and happy in his flat.
- The conditions of his flat were not of an acceptable standard.
- He felt as if decisions were being made 'about' him and he began to distrust people.
- He declined the support of some agencies and was reluctant to engage with others.
- He felt out of control of his life and he said to his niece on two occasions that he felt like a burden and he wanted to die.

At the end of the review, the niece gave her view on what should have happened, which included:

- for Derek to have been asked what he wanted rather than be told;
- for her to have been able to ask for support and contribute with Derek to a plan that would have made Derek feel happy and in control;
- for his housing situation to have been addressed;
- for all the agencies to have got together and for someone to take the lead;
- for agencies to have recognised how ill Derek felt and how this was significantly impacting his mental health and his quality of life.

The report stated:

Professional curiosity was not always evident and assessments, particularly in the hospital context and discharge processes, relied heavily on self-report, with home circumstances not observed and family members or general practice staff not consulted.

(Berry, 2022, p 11, section 8.2.6)

REFLECTIVE QUESTIONS

- Drawing from the four types of listeners, identify how each could impact your engagement with others.
- Using Table 1.1 in Chapter 1, identify which skills and attributes could support professional curiosity practice. Think about Derek's experience and how those skills might have changed his experience.

In relation to Derek, the findings from the review suggest, as you may have identified, the importance of empathy in safeguarding practice, including the ability to understand the person's perspective of risk and what is important to them. Another factor might have been openness and honesty. The report suggests that Derek began to distrust people because he was not being included or involved – because decisions were being made about him without him (Berry, 2022).

Trauma-informed practice and professional curiosity: asking 'why?'

The impact of trauma (either from specific events or the longer-term impact of experiences, such as neglect or witnessing domestic or other abuse) is increasingly being recognised as an important factor when working with children and adults. People's responses to certain situations have often been formed through past experiences (perhaps where they felt frightened, humiliated, unsafe, trapped, ashamed, powerless, rejected or unsupported) and can be automatic reactions by people to keep themselves safe. There is much research on the impact of adverse childhood experiences (Asmussen et al, 2020) and, often when reviews involving adults are undertaken, traumatic experiences will be identified that provide context for why someone behaved the way they did, made certain choices, did not 'engage' with professionals or refused support. So, trauma-informed practice in simple terms means being aware of the impact trauma may have had, or be having, using your curiosity to think of and explore what may have happened in the past and responding accordingly. To return to the point above about over-professionalising concepts, it is not about providing therapy, but rather developing trust, meaningful relationships and engagement with the individual, all with the intention of preventing harm. This includes looking to prevent secondary trauma, where an intervention simply compounds and reinforces negative experiences.

Northumberland's Child Safeguarding Practice Review (CSPR) of Sophia (MacDonald, 2024) uses appreciative enquiry and reports in the first person (the voice of the child), identifying strengths and successes while recognising the impact of trauma not only on Sophia but on the network around her. The report references the Office for Health Improvement and Disparities (OHID, 2022) Guidance: Working Definition of Trauma-informed Practice and reminds us that a trauma-informed approach 'requires people to look beyond "behaviours" to ask what does the child need rather than what is wrong with them'. A key learning point in this review is, once again, the need to share information between agencies and use curiosity.

In another case review, the Rotherham SAR 'The Painter and His Son', there were some notable examples of good practice in relation to professional curiosity and recognising trauma (Spreadbury, 2021). The Painter, Sam, was found dead in April 2019 at age 91 (he had potentially been dead for many weeks). His son, Ben, was 61 when he was found a year later, also having been deceased for several months, his cause of death therefore unascertainable.

Following Sam's death, the social worker recounted that:

> *The first time she met him he was shaking, and she wondered if this was acute alcohol withdrawal. He was pleasant but 'stand-offish' and she felt conscious of*

being 'in his space'. He initially did not engage, and it was thought that he must be experiencing trauma. He seemed embarrassed that he had let 'things get like this'.

(Spreadbury, 2021, p 19, 4.9)

The report indicates that:

Social workers demonstrated good practice, working with Ben, observing his needs and reactions as best they could as well as using their professional curiosity to respectfully challenge Ben and try to understand his experiences. Unanswered telephone calls were followed up with unannounced visits, Ben could have no doubt that social workers were concerned about him and ready to support him.

(Spreadbury, 2021, p 26, 4.12)

Workers in this case showed an awareness of the traumatic impact of Ben's experiences, particularly in terms of his ability to engage/communicate, and were persistent and consistent in approach (Spreadbury, 2021). While learning from SARs seeks to drive further improvement in practice, even this will not always change the final outcome; however, in some cases it will, and using professional curiosity to consider the complexities of an adult's situation and experience can at least maximise opportunities for positive change and engagement.

APPLYING CONCEPTS TO PRACTICE

Case study

Malcolm and Emma have been married for nearly 60 years. They have lived independently until the last six months, when Emma was diagnosed with an advanced cancer. Malcom has become her main carer. An occupational therapist (OT) has been to visit and is now raising safeguarding concerns because Malcolm has built a piece of equipment to move Emma upstairs, which the OT believes is not safe. He is also refusing to have a hospital bed downstairs, or an air mattress that will help to prevent her skin from breaking down. Emma is asleep much of the time and at the moment her skin is intact. Malcolm got angry with the OT during the visit and asked her to leave – he will not allow them back in the house.

TASK

- Write down at least four possible reasons why Malcom might be responding in this way.
- Which of your professional curiosity skills would you use when engaging with Malcolm and Emma, and why?

Effective practice skills

In the case scenario relating to Malcolm, mentioned above, the OT is now working with social worker Martina. She initially assessed the potential risk to Emma as high due to the use of potentially dangerous equipment, and decided to do an unannounced visit as it was very likely that Malcolm would refuse an arranged one. However, she had also considered some possible reasons for Malcolm being so angry:

- Malcolm may be struggling in his role as a carer;
- he may be feeling undermined by the professionals coming into their home;
- he could be controlling and restricting access to Emma.

Martina reflected before the visit that she was feeling anxious and worried that Malcolm might become angry towards her too. She thought about what she would say on arrival, and about keeping her body language as well as her words relaxed, non-judgemental and supportive. As she arrived, she took some deep breaths to calm herself down and smiled as he opened the door. Martina used her planned communication skills and empathy to explain to Malcolm that she wanted to do a general review of how he and Emma were doing, to hear his views about the help they might need. She allowed him time to talk about their day-to-day routine, which gave her the chance to look at the equipment he was using and explore the risks to Emma.

Using gentle probing and open questions, she found out more about his caring role, his views on the equipment and his relationships with professionals coming into their home. Through this, she determined that Malcolm felt his ability to care was being questioned and he was not seen as the expert on his wife's needs. He clearly stated that he wanted to care for her to the end of her life and that he had promised her she would never have to go into a care home. It was also evident that he had been thinking about what the OT had said and had been reading information the community nurses had left him, so he was more open to the idea of the equipment proposed. Martina realised that Malcolm needed time to process change, and if rushed he became defensive and responded angrily because of this. She was able to share that information with the OT and nurses, to make their engagements with Malcolm more positive and effective too.

In this case, the professional views on the risks were very much preventative, as no actual harm had occurred. Taking the time to learn what lay behind Malcolm's responses, working together and giving him time to process information all meant intervention was possible. Malcolm could continue caring safely, and Emma was able to die in her own home.

Making 'unwise choices' and professional curiosity

As mentioned, professional curiosity is noted as a theme in SARs and other reviews, and often in relation to the adult making 'unwise choices' – perhaps declining support and intervention from the people trying to work with them. The link may be that an assumption of capacity meant that the 'why' wasn't explored, that agencies withdrew support or did not share information in a multi-agency forum (Jones, 2022). In the SAR of Derek (Berry, 2022) mentioned above, he did have a learning disability, but the review noted he '*worked during parts of his earlier life and functioned quite independently with support required in some aspects of his life*' (Berry, 2022, p 6, 6.1). This relative independence may have supported assumptions being made about his mental capacity. However, the review found that:

> *There is lots of evidence that there were known risk factors across the agencies and with more robust professional curiosity should have led to questions about Derek's ability to make certain decisions at certain times … This review found that there was an absence of professional curiosity that resulted in inaction rather than action.*
>
> (Berry, 2022, pp 13, 8.3.6 and 22, 9.23)

Chapter 3 explored the concept of cognitive bias and considered its impact on professional curiosity. In Derek's case, the evidence of his independent living led to assumptions about his mental capacity and in particular his executive functioning (we will explore mental capacity and what is meant by executive function in Chapter 5), dulling the need to ask more questions. You might think of this in terms of checking that a person can 'walk the walk' simply by asking 'show me'. Is what you see the same as what you are being told? In Rochdale Adult L (Sandiford, 2023a), a learning event was held and those present suggested that the lack of visual evidence impacted professional curiosity about how she was managing. The review said:

> *For example, if a visiting professional had been told by Adult L that she was managing but could see that she was looking unclean and unkempt, the professional would pose further questions. Similarly, when professionals spoke with Adult L through the window, they lost any visual triggers regarding home conditions.*
>
> (Sandiford, 2023a, p 15, 7.40)

The concept of what is or isn't an unwise choice is arguably the most open to wide interpretation. The point being made is that someone would not automatically lack capacity simply on another person's judgement about their decisions – taking risks, for example – so it is not quite the same as 'having a right to make unwise choices', which suggests a subtext of 'we can't intervene'.

The SAR of Adult K commissioned by Teeside Safeguarding Adult Board (Sahota, 2023) considered the circumstances of a non-fatal fire in the home of an adult with needs related to their mental health and the subsequent impact of that fire on the person. Key themes were the interface between mental health and mental capacity, linked to self-neglect (Sahota, 2023). Adult K insisted that they were going to clean and tidy their environment, refusing external support, but concerns about their home continued to the point where a serious fire occurred. The reviewer said, '*the practitioners should have been prompted to assess Adult K's executive capacity by their refusals of aid and claims to care for their property'* (Sahota, 2023, p 5, 3.15). Similarly in Wokingham, the SAR of Tina (Whitehead, 2023) involved an adult who was admitted to hospital severely emaciated, with muscle wastage and skin damage. She had been sleeping/living on the sofa for five months prior to her hospital admission. She died five days later, aged 83. Her husband had been her main carer. Tina had declined intervention and offers of equipment to support her needs over a long period of time. The house was noted as 'hoarded', with evidence of self-neglect. She also had a history and more recent indicators of alcohol dependency. The review found that the reasons behind her declining support were not explored by some of the agencies involved. Her mental capacity was not questioned as she had no evident cognitive impairment, even with the escalating risks to her health and well-being. Her refusals of help became normalised.

Through the review, Tina's daughter advised that her mother had been drinking heavily up to two weeks before she died. When a physiotherapist visited:

> *A bottle of red wine was observed on the table, Tina stated she had one glass a day. There was no further questions or professional curiosity on Tina's alcohol intake, no consideration given to the impact alcohol may have on Tina's ability to make decisions*
>
> (Whitehead, 2023, p 6)

There was also limited use of multi-agency discussions/meetings or planning as her physical condition deteriorated. The review also noted that opportunities were missed to explore Tina's husband's needs and views as her main carer – to support him and also potentially understand Tina's decision-making, given the high levels of risk identified (Whitehead, 2023, p 11). This highlights the value of not just dealing with the presenting issue, as to do so can miss the needs of carers, or other factors that are likely to have a high impact.

Another example of this can be seen in the Norfolk DHR for Daisy (Mears, 2020). In this case Daisy had a range of physical health needs and no impairment to her capacity, but was very dependent on her husband as her main carer. His own needs were generally subsumed by the focus on Daisy, with little curiosity or support about his developing dementia. This led to a situation where his misunderstanding of the purpose of her respite care meant he killed her and then tried to take his own life (Mears, 2020).

In the SAR of Tina (above), there were some examples of good practice (see below), but it was not consistent throughout the period of the review, as noted in the SAR report:

> *In October 2022 the visit from the Community Matron respected Tina's wishes but continued to revisit the decision regarding going to hospital until Tina agreed. Tina's longstanding wishes of not wanting to be admitted to hospital were respected for as long as possible. The Community Matron correctly raised a safeguarding referral from her visit and completed Datix. There was clear evidence of professional curiosity demonstrated.*
>
> (Whitehead, 2023, p 11)

REFLECTIVE QUESTIONS

- Thinking about the enablers of professional curiosity discussed in Chapter 3 and the tips to support holding difficult conversations, how might you use these in Tina's case?

The impact of power

Situations of safeguarding usually involve the abuse of power that one person has over another. Family and other interpersonal relationships can be highly complex so using your curiosity to understand where power sits around any particular decision or behaviour may give you more opportunity to challenge or rebalance, potentially enabling the adult to hold more control over their life and preventing further abuse. In the Nottinghamshire SAR about Adult C (Frame, 2017), the report notes that Adult C was 'protective of his abusers' and that a lack of professional curiosity meant the impact of coercion and control was not considered in relation to his inability to engage with agencies. It is important to know that trauma can be a factor where someone is being emotionally controlled.

REFLECTIVE QUESTIONS

Think of a domestic abuser deliberately threatening to leave an adult who has experienced profound grief and/or loss in the past, in the knowledge the person will remember those negative feelings from the past and beg them to stay. What would you do in this context?

This is also a good example of how trauma can have an impact executive functioning. In this context, the response is not reasoned as such, but an automatic response triggered by past experience.

Professional curiosity in a multi-agency context

In the Rotherham SAR mentioned previously (The Painter and His Son), one of the learning points said:

> Staff [Adult Social Care] were using a professionally curious approach when working with Ben but could not explore their understanding fully without access to partner colleagues' expertise to help them unpick some of the challenges they experienced.

(Spreadbury, 2021, p 29)

The phrase 'safeguarding is everybody's business' is used for a reason. In terms of both prevention and statutory enquiry, safeguarding involves adults in our communities who often need or are in receipt of some kind of service, meaning that there will usually be connections with a variety of different people and agencies, holding different amounts or types of information. Most retrospective reviews will identify examples of where information has not been shared, or people not involved, where that could have made a significant difference to the experiences or outcomes for the adult or child. Having a rounded, holistic understanding of a person can support better engagement, more effective interventions and improved outcomes. It is also clear that professional curiosity is not limited to those with 'professional' in their job title – anyone may feel that something isn't quite right, and have that gut instinct or other cognitive niggle that prompts them to ask more questions. Those questions may not always be directly to the adult or child – but sharing with peers or in a multi-agency collaboration setting (for example) may be the first point of applying that curious thinking.

Think the unthinkable – in the Local Safeguarding Practice Review of Baby Y (Doherty, 2024), which considered non-accidental injuries to a nine-month old baby, while there was much positive comment about the relationship built up by the health visitor with Baby Y's mum, there was concern about the lack of enquiry about the dad or the new partner, Adult A (the latter was found to be the perpetrator of the abuse) and that the health visitor ended up working in some isolation:

> *An issue that emerged for practitioners who contributed to the review was about how to work with uncertainty and 'gut feeling'. The health visitor felt that much of what Mother reported about Adult A was suspicious, but this in itself did not amount to a safeguarding concern. This is a familiar dilemma in multi-agency safeguarding work and resonated with those who took part in the learning event. Practitioners felt that without hard evidence and factual information, they were much less likely to escalate their concerns. Moreover, concerns born mainly from gut instinct were less likely to be accepted into other services such as Early Help and front door services in social care.*

(Doherty, 2024, 6.13)

The review promoted the use of supervision as a reflective space to work through those gut feelings in a more analytical and evidenced way, to support the legitimacy of them. It stated as a key finding:

> *Gut instinct and professional curiosity are important aspects of multi-agency work that should not be underestimated. Both of these should be given airtime to discuss.*

(Doherty, 2024, 6.14)

The review did identify some really good practice noted about the relationship built up by the health visitor, who got to know the family very well, with a good rapport established. The worker was noted as '*keen to work in partnership*', working alongside the family to support changes – but was also working in isolation as she wasn't quite sure how to escalate her concerns which may not have met thresholds for safeguarding (Doherty, 2024).

Professional difficulties and escalating concerns

Where multiple agencies are involved in cases involving adults or families, reviews show us over and over again how important good communication is, to ensure everyone has the same information in order to enable effective and holistic risk assessment and management and to develop the appropriate and proportionate actions needed to ultimately achieve positive outcomes for the individuals in need of support. One challenge in multi-agency forums can be that some people or organisations may seem to have a stronger voice, or a more 'valid' opinion, potentially based on simply having a more formal title, qualification or senior role. This runs the risk of others feeling invalidated, dismissed or just ignored – which can lead to frustration, anger or disengagement. Most importantly for the subject of the discussion, it can mean that different perspectives and risks are not accurately considered, potential bias and judgement is not challenged, and those agencies will be reluctant to participate in future.

One way to address this is through skilled chairing of such meetings. For example, if you are the Chair, consider whether you have made sure everyone around the table has had an equal opportunity to give their view. Do the notes/minutes accurately reflect what was said, what was agreed and why? Did anyone have a differing view and how is that recorded?

As a participant, you can insist that your view is recorded, and/or put your concern in writing to the Chair. Outside of meetings, where you feel uncomfortable or continue to be concerned about an adult or a child, clearly record your concerns as factually as you can, ask for specific reasons why something is or is not being done, look at what escalation processes you have access to. Speak to your manager or check what your local SAB offers in terms of those pathways where the concerns are specific to safeguarding.

Real examples of professional curiosity in different settings

In all the following examples, the person using their curiosity was not a 'professional', but they used their curiosity and took those next steps to find out 'why' something had happened.

An autistic young adult who also had ADHD was living with a family member – their household moved into temporary accommodation and then moved again to a different address. A bill came to the temporary address, so the new tenants there handed it to their local council tenancy team to pass on. The council officer contacted the family member, who asked them to open the letter, which was found to be a utility bill in the names of both the family member (the tenant) and the young adult. It was a large bill, in arrears, and the letter advised that legal action may be taken.

At this point the worker could have moved on – they weren't being asked to do anything else and didn't have a specific responsibility to the young adult. However, using their professional curiosity, the officer considered various concerns, and went to discuss with their safeguarding lead. The concerns identified were:

- the young adult shouldn't have been named on the utility bill (they were not the actual tenant);
- would they have the mental capacity to understand what being on the bill meant?
- they were worried about the young adult's liability for the bill and potential legal action if there was insufficient understanding;
- there was concern about possible financial abuse – questions about how the person's money was being used as their benefit payments went directly into the family member's bank account.

Looking at the information the council held on the individuals, they saw past conversations with the young person about finances as they were keen to have their own home, but a reluctance to talk in detail about their money, saying that their family member did it all and that is what they wanted. Records showed that other family members had always managed the money – but it was unclear whether that was related to the young adult's mental capacity or their practical ability/desire to manage themselves. Being curious meant that records were checked and supportive discussions were held within the housing team and with the safeguarding lead. This led to a safeguarding concern being raised to the local authority so further enquiries could be made.

In another example, a member of local council staff was delivering leaflets in an area and noticed one house with an overgrown garden, curtains drawn and mail piled up behind the door to the point where they couldn't get the leaflet through the letterbox. The worker was just delivering leaflets, and was not sure what else to do, but continued to feel concerned. When they got back to their office, they decided to speak to their safeguarding lead, which led to a check on council tax records for any other indicators of concern. This didn't find anything, but the safeguarding lead supported the worker's wish to follow up with a phone call. They spoke to the occupier, who was fine and explained the post build up – the person was actually very appreciative of the call and thanked the worker for checking that they were okay. The worker also felt reassured that they had done the right thing.

In a further example, a woman came into a library with a black eye, looking upset and wanting to use a computer. One of the library assistants helped with this and asked whether she needed any other help, but she said she was okay. The staff member was still concerned, and after a bit more conversation managed to find out that the woman had been attacked by someone living at the site she was staying on. She had fled for safety with no money or phone. The staff member said she would speak to the library manager and try to help. After hearing the concerns, the manager came to speak to her, and said the woman had mental health needs and had tried to end her life in the past. She wanted to speak to someone as she was concerned she was going to try and kill herself again because she didn't know what to do and felt alone and scared. She said she was now homeless because she couldn't go back to the site as she was too frightened. She had no money to get to family elsewhere in the country and became upset again, saying she felt 'hopeless'.

She was offered help to report the attack and her injuries to the police, but she said it would make things worse. The library staff tried a local crisis team but were unable to get through – they then contacted a local community project, which in turn contacted the local council to provide support with accommodation and accessing mental health support. The council offices were close by, so the library staff walked there with the woman and waited until the emergency housing officer arrived. They checked with her that she was now okay to be left, after confirming that she would be supported to get the help she needed. Here is a useful quote from the library manager:

> *She told me on the walk over that she didn't know what she would have done if I hadn't helped but she didn't think it would have been good. I asked her what made her come to the library this morning and she said she had been in before and we were always really kind. She was walking down the road and saw the building and just decided to come in, so she felt safe.*
>
> (PWLE, anonymised)

Practice tips

Keep the person central – an example from the seven-minute briefing for the SAR about John (West Berkshire Safeguarding Adult Board, 2023) makes the point that although it is important to respect autonomy and self-determination, professional curiosity helps the triangulation of information, in turn maintaining a healthier balance between the views of others and the direct contact/assessment of the person themselves. Think family – who else is involved with the person? Where you have a specific role with an individual, or purpose for a visit, remember to be curious about others around them. You may be the only person who has been into the property, so the only person in a position to use that curiosity. Or you may be the first one of many visitors who actually does notice a carer, the child, the friend and ask questions that others may have missed. In the SAR of Gaynor (Tameside Adults Safeguarding Partnership Board, 2023) the case involved a complex family situation, multiple needs (including concerns around self-neglect), and a variety of professionals involved. The review states:

> *Whilst it was clear that concerns were raised about Gaynor's physical and mental health, there was little regard made to considering that Gaynor was a vulnerable adult herself or the impact which any health difficulties identified would have on her ability to care for others. Despite clear evidence, prompted by disclosures being made by (family), safeguarding of the family was fragmented and opportunities were missed in ensuring that the family was safe.*
>
> (Tameside Adults Safeguarding Partnership Board, 2023, p 11)

It is important to recognise where work pressures are affecting your curiosity, including pressure to close cases or discontinue interventions. Burton and Revell (2018) identified how the impact of a stressful work environment on workers reduces capacity to check history, challenge or ask questions.

What systems barriers do you need to be aware of? For example, the majority of systems are mostly available during working hours. In the SAR of Adult C, Frame (2017, para 5.2) notes that the adult

> *presented to very many professionals over the scoping period of this review but mainly in connection with an immediate need – for example, needing shelter, and mostly at night, so was supported by out of hours services.*

Adult C also moved between authority boundaries. The SAR report commented that *'his health, housing and social care needs were never fully met'* (Frame, 2017, para 5.2). In complex cases, there may be a large amount of information to read for background, and sometimes information technology (IT) systems make this harder, perhaps because of the way information is set out or because they don't talk to each other (see, for example, Norfolk SAR L, M and N and SAR Sonia in Kent and Medway (Nicholls, 2022).

Make the most of any 'window of opportunity'. The SAR of Adult L (Sandiford, 2023a) reminds us that individual consent can be overridden if professional curiosity identifies risk of significant harm, and urges using every possible chance to engage where opportunities are otherwise infrequent. Further, when those windows did not appear, the review noted that it was *'imperative that professionals consulted each other, and historic case notes, in an attempt to understand Adult L better'* (Sandiford, 2023a, p 13).

REFLECTIVE QUESTIONS

Think about any biases you may hold – our own values and beliefs are shaped through our individual social development and experiences, often mirroring those of the people we learn from most directly (family, close friends, teachers) as well as the groups in society we feel we belong most to, potentially reinforced by the algorithms of social media.

- How might these influence your curiosity about the people you work to support?
- How aware are you of different cultural norms, of how these may change a person's presentation or behaviour?
- Would you think to ask a male if he feels safe at home in the same way that you might make such a routine enquiry of a female? If not, why not?

In the SAR of Adult C, it was noted that professional assumptions (were) made as a result of diagnostic labels and gender bias in relation to a homeless young man, who had a history of mental health and substance misuse problems, presenting with injuries and explanations that matched a stereotypical view of him (Frame, 2017). He was not seen as someone at increased risk/with additional vulnerabilities because of his homeless status. Multidisciplinary working and decision-making can help challenge bias – it can open out your perspective and thinking, asking the 'why' of each other, forming a more rounded view of an adult, their situation or decisions.

REFLECTIVE QUESTIONS

Think about assumption and bias, particularly in relation to non-engagement (people who don't attend appointments).

- What might your instinctive responses be to someone aged 77 with a diagnosis of dementia who is refusing intervention, compared with someone in their early twenties who is dependent on drugs or alcohol and refusing help?
- Why might that change your own personal instinct to be curious about why they refuse?

The concept of adultification was introduced in Chapter 2. As mentioned, adultification revolves around a perception that a child is more adult in their specific behaviour or presentation, which feeds an assumption that they are not as vulnerable or innocent. The Case of Child F (Botham, 2024) draws attention to the impact of adultification when working with those at risk of criminal and/or sexual exploitation. Citing Davis and Marsh (2020), Davis (2022, p 5) notes that *'this is determined by people and institutions who hold power over them* [the child] *and when adultification occurs outside of the home it is always founded within discrimination and bias'*.

Child F was a child in local authority care who experienced a traumatic and possibly targeted assault linked to criminal exploitation, leaving him with life-changing injuries. The review found that the contextual and safeguarding risks he was subject to, including exploitation, had generally not been recognised or responded to by the range of agencies involved with him. Adultification was cited as a specific barrier to professional curiosity in this case.

This provides a good example of how this might be reflected in the language you use with different people (para 3.14):

- sofa surfing as opposed to homeless;
- did not attend as opposed to was not brought;
- making unhealthy choices, choosing to drug deal;
- 'streetwise', as opposed to potentially being exploited;
- inappropriate relationship rather than abuse of power.

> ### REFLECTIVE QUESTION
>
> Phillips et al (2024) describe using professional curiosity as 'opening Pandora's Box', with potentially difficult feelings associated. Examples include asking 'Can I handle this?' and 'What will I do?'
>
> - Write down what helps you to stay curious when you feel like this.

Some examples might be planning well; reminding yourself of the purpose of the questions/visit; remembering your duty of care; and knowing it's okay not to be okay, and also okay to ask for help.

Starting difficult conversations is important – using your professional curiosity is not simply a tick-box exercise. You will have been in situations yourself where you have been asked a question and you know very well the person asking it has no real interest in the answer, but they have been told to ask it, or feel they must do so. You are then much more likely to answer with a brief or stock reply because you know instinctively that the person doesn't have a real interest.

There is a key lesson in being curious: mean it. Be genuine, be honest. The second key thing (and this is arguably harder) is to have time – how many times do you say to friends or colleagues 'You alright?' as a polite query while rushing past or hoping they don't have too much to reply with. In that kind of scenario, you are more likely not to even ask and, being busy, more likely not to listen to the answer.

It is fine to have a stock opening/open question, as long as the follow-up interaction is individualised. For example:

- How are things at home?
- Is there anything worrying you at the moment?
- Tell me what things you worry most about.
- You sound like you have a lot going on at the moment – how you are really feeling?
- You're really giving a lot of help to X – how is that affecting you?

> ### KEY POINTS FROM THIS CHAPTER
>
> - Be curious whatever your role – you don't need to consider yourself a 'professional' to use curiosity in your working day, or as part of your community – be interested and ask questions. Safeguarding is everybody's business.

- SARs, CSPRs and DARDRs give us the chance to look back in depth at the points in people's lives where doing something differently might have changed the outcome for the adult or child – they help you to learn lessons and adapt your working practice to prevent abuse and/or neglect in future.
- Professional curiosity is a regular theme in such reviews, most usually where it has not been used; recognise the value of multi-agency collaboration, working together to create a full and accurate picture of the adult or child you are all there to support.
- Keep the adult central to everything you do; be aware of your own attitudes to risk or cultural bias and have the confidence to challenge or engage with others where you feel a voice is going unheard.

Further reading

Organisation for Security and Co-operation in Europe (OSCE) and Office for Democratic Institutions and Human Rights (ODIHR) (2023) *Guidance on Trauma-informed National Referral Mechanisms and Responses to Human Trafficking*. [online] Available at: www.osce.org/files/f/documents/1/9/549793.pdf (accessed 13 November 2024).

This provides guidance on trauma-informed practice.

5 The legal and policy context of partnership work in safeguarding adults

CHAPTER OBJECTIVES

By end of this chapter, you should be able to:

- understand what is meant by partnership working in safeguarding practice;
- ascertain the importance of partnership work in safeguarding adult work;
- understand the legal and policy context of partnership work in safeguarding adult practice;
- use the knowledge gained to inform participation in professional curiosity practice when working with those at risk of or who are experiencing abuse, harm and neglect.

Introduction

This chapter focuses on the legal and policy context of partnership work in safeguarding adult work. It considers partnership working between different agencies engaged in safeguarding adult work as well as the partnership between practitioners and individuals at risk of or experiencing abuse, harm and neglect, their families and carers in professional curiosity practice. The chapter begins by examining the concept of partnership working and why partnership work is important in safeguarding adult work.

What is partnership work?

Partnership working is embedded in safeguarding adult practice as a key policy initiative across the United Kingdom. It is achieved through joint working (integration of health and social care), cooperation and collaboration. The term is often used interchangeably within the literature with multi-agency/inter-agency working, interprofessional/interdisciplinary working and integration. Percy-Smith (2006, p 316) notes that partnership working occurs in '*any situation in which people work across organisational boundaries towards some positive end*'. More recently, Fynn et al (2022, p 286) used the concept of partnership work '*to describe any context in which two or more actors interact for the purposes of their work*'. In safeguarding adult work, we use multi-agency, interprofessional and interdisciplinary work to facilitate effective joint working to allow organisations to work in partnership with each other in the best interests of those who are at risk of abuse or have experienced abuse. Partnership working brings different practitioners from diverse backgrounds and professions together so different expertise and resources are pulled together to support those at risk or experiencing abuse, neglect and harm. The literature identifies different models of partnership working, including an economically driven model, a learning culture model and person-centred partnership work. Literature examining the different types of partnership work suggest the economically driven partnership model limits the potential for all parties to participate on equal terms (eg people who use services). Person-centred partnership working allows '*the production of intelligent, flexible services with a high degree of client participation*'. Person-centred partnership work extends the scope to include all partners, including those at the centre of safeguarding concern; it fosters collegiality by enabling all partners to work together to maximise positive outcomes for people at the centre of care. The learning partnership model encourages reflexivity and learning (Fynn et al, 2022). Table 5.1 provides characteristics that lead to effective partnership and processes that you might find useful. Engagement in professional curiosity practice assists us to critically evaluate the context, the environment, input (resources), skills, expertise and processes (eg activities such as systems of referrals and decision-making processes) within partnership and collaborative working practices to ensure that resources are used effectively to make people safe.

Why is partnership working important in safeguarding work?

In the United Kingdom and internationally, agencies from the public, private, independent and voluntary sectors are obligated by policy and law to work together to identify, and find solutions to prevent, minimise, mitigate, stop and protect, people suffering from abuse, harm and neglect (DHSC, 2024; WHO, 2021). As well as working with other professionals, effective partnership work obliges practitioners to work collaboratively with the people who are at risk of abuse, their families and carers. However, safeguarding adult reviews (SARs) have repeatedly cited a lack of partnership working and joined-up working, as well as a lack of cooperation between professionals and agencies in the enquiries into the deaths of adults and children (Preston-Shoot et al, 2024; Thacker et al, 2019). The SAR relating to Brian commissioned by Swindon Safeguarding Partnership Board (Hopkinson, 2023) provides one example of why joined-up working and professional curiosity are important in safeguarding work.

> **APPLYING CONCEPTS TO PRACTICE**
>
> Case study
>
> The importance of professional curiosity and partnership work – the human story
>
> > Brian was a 43-year-old white British man who had mental health needs and a history of drug use. He lived alone in a flat, where he died in a fire on 7 February 2022. From July 2020 until his death, Brian was in contact with several agencies including the police, the ambulance service, mental and physical health services, and specialist drug services in response to self-neglect and drug dependency. Agencies struggled to engage with Brian who spent periods of time away from his flat, staying in hotels. Brian had mental health needs and a long history of poly-substance misuse, particularly heroin and cannabis, with alcohol misuse also noted.
> >
> > (Hopkinson, 2023, p 3)
>
> Hopkinson (2023, p 29, 7.1, 7.2) notes that
>
> > there was no coordinated multi-agency response to Brian's needs. These could have enabled all the agencies to pool their knowledge of Brian. This may have resulted in the generation of new and coordinated support.
>
> The SAR on Brian draws attention to the human story of why professional curiosity and partnership working are important in safeguarding those at risk of harm, abuse and neglect (Hopkinson, 2023). You have an important role to play in working with others to ensure no one comes to harm.

REFLECTIVE QUESTIONS

- What are your thoughts in relation to the SAR of Brian?
- Why do you think partnership working is important in this case?
- Thinking about the models of partnership working introduced earlier, what model would you use to ensure effective partnership with all involved?
- How would you use professional curiosity in the context of this work?
- What curious questions would you ask and why?
- What learning would you take forward to inform your future practice?

Table 5.1 *Characteristics that lead to effective partnership and processes*

- Compassionate listening
- Perspective listening
- Regular communication and continuity
- Establishing clear goals and outcomes including risk and escalation plans
- Modelling professional curiosity
- Effective monitoring of needs risks and risk-enablement plans
- Involvement of people who use services in risk identification and risk-enablement plans
- Trust
- Honesty
- Transparency
- Resilience
- High levels of engagement, accountability and feedback
- Knowledge exchange and capacity-building
- Information-sharing and expertise
- Sharing of resources and experience for mutual benefit
- Co-creation of the production of knowledge
- Professional courage and learning

Source: The summary has been drawn from Anka (2023), Flynn et al (2022), Lawless et al (2020), Miller et al (2021).

The legal framework for safeguarding adults with a specific focus on partnership work in the UK

Safeguarding adult legislation varies across the four constituted countries of the United Kingdom (England, Wales, Northern Ireland and Scotland, please see Table 5.3). Differences exist in the definitions of those to whom protection and safeguarding is due. Due to this, approaches to safeguarding adults across the four constituted countries of the United Kingdom also differ. Although these differences exist, all the legislative frameworks in the four constituted countries of the United Kingdom reinforce partnership working achieved through effective joined working and cooperation between agencies. What follows looks at the legislative context of safeguarding adult work in the four countries of the United Kingdom with a specific focus on partnership working.

England

The *Care Act 2014* is the main legislative framework for safeguarding adults in England. The 2014 Act sets out the legal mandate for local authorities to work with others to protect people from harm, abuse and neglect through the development of Safeguarding Adult Boards (SABs). The main safeguarding adult duties under the *Care Act 2014* are contained in sections 42–47. The statutory guidance accompanying the *Care Act 2014* (DHSC, 2024, 14.7) specifies that safeguarding adults requires '*people and organisations working together to prevent and stop both the risks and experience of abuse or neglect*'. Another section of the Act, section 3, focuses on integration of social care and healthcare services while sections 6 and 7 focus on cooperation. Under section 6 of the *Care Act 2014*, local authorities have a duty to cooperate with other agencies; they can also request others to cooperate with them under section 7. The statutory guidance accompanying the *Care Act 2014* (DHSC, 2024, 14.17) defines a range of factors that constitute abuse to include:

- physical abuse;
- domestic violence;
- sexual abuse;
- psychological abuse;
- financial or material abuse;
- modern slavery;
- discriminatory abuse;
- organisational abuse;
- neglect and acts of omission;
- self-neglect.

The statutory guidance (DHSC, 2024) makes clear that you should not limit your views of what constitutes abuse and neglect, as abuse can take many forms.

The role of Safeguarding Adult Boards

The *Care Act 2014* provides the strategic infrastructure for local authorities and its partner agencies to work together to safeguard adults. Section 43 mandates local authorities to establish SABs for its area. The SAB has the strategic overview to develop and then execute safeguarding plans to help and protect adults in its area from abuse, harm and neglect through coordinating and effective multi-agency partnership working. The membership of a SAB includes local authorities, police and integrated care board as statutory partners. Under section 44(1), (2), (3), (4) and (5) of the *Care Act 2014*, SABs are required to arrange a Safeguarding Adult Review (SAR) where an adult with care and support needs dies or an adult has experienced serious harm, abuse or neglect and there are concerns about how agencies worked together to safeguard the adult in order to identify what can be learnt so as to apply the lessons to future cases to prevent harm and abuse. SABs are also mandated to request information from practitioners under section 45 of the *Care Act 2014*. Although the main duties of safeguarding adults under the *Care Act 2014* are contained under sections 42–47, other sections of the Act may apply depending upon the individual circumstances and in line with the threshold criterion set by the *Care Act 2014*, as explained in the following section.

Safeguarding adult duties under section 42 of the *Care Act 2014*

Section 42 duties exist at the point where safeguarding concerns are raised. Local authorities are required to make enquiries or cause others to do so on their behalf when they suspect that an adult with care and support needs is at risk of, or experiencing, abuse and neglect, and where, because of the care and support needs, the adult is unable to protect themselves. There is a two-stage process within section 42. The first stage is an information-gathering stage and has a strong focus on prevention. Practitioners are required to gather information at this stage to ascertain whether the safeguarding concerns meet section 42(1) criteria:

Section 42(1) of the Care Act 2014, safeguarding duties, applies to an adult who:

(a) *has needs for care and support (whether or not the local authority is meeting any of those needs);*

(b) *is experiencing, or at risk of, abuse or neglect;*

(c) *as a result of those care and support needs is unable to protect themselves from either the risk of, or the experience of abuse or neglect.*

Once established that there is reasonable cause to suspect that the adult meets the section 42(1) *Care Act 2014* criteria (as above), then a section 42(2) duty is triggered:

Under section 42(2) of the Care Act 2014, local authorities:

(a) *must make (or cause to be made) whatever enquiries are necessary;*

(b) *decide whether any action should be taken in the adult's case and, if so, what and by whom.*

Practitioners are also obligated to draw from other sections of the *Care Act 2014* to inform practice. Prevention and well-being are core principles underpinning the *Care Act 2014* and are central to safeguarding adults. When exercising your public duties under the Act, you are obligated to promote the well-being of adults at risk of harm, abuse and neglect. Section 1(2) of the *Care Act 2014* provides a well-being checklist that you must use to inform their assessments as follows:

(a) *personal dignity (including treatment of the individual with respect);*

(b) *physical and mental health and emotional wellbeing;*

(c) protection from abuse and neglect;

(d) control by the individual over day-to-day life (including over care and support, or support, provided to the individual and the way in which it is provided);

(e) participation in work, education, training or recreation;

(f) social and economic wellbeing;

(g) domestic, family and personal relationships;

(h) suitability of living accommodation;

(i) the individual's contribution to society.

The *Care Act 2014* requires you to use strengths-based and person-centred approaches to engage with those who are experiencing or at risk of harm, abuse and neglect. Section 1(3)(b) of the Act stipulates that you must include the adults' views, wishes, feelings and beliefs in the safeguarding assessment and interventions. You are also obligated to provide information and advice under section 4 to enable people to take part in decision-making processes. The information and advice provided should be accessible, and proportionate to the needs of those for whom they are being provided. Further, sections 9 and 10 obligate local authorities to carry out a needs assessment of the adult and a carer's assessment respectively. It is important to remember that under section 9(3)(a) and (b) and section 10)(4)(a) and (b), every adult and every carer respectively has a legal right to an assessment, regardless of the level of care and support needed and regardless of the level of financial resources they may have. The *Care Act* also mandates the involvement of people with care and support needs in assessment under section 9(5) and carers under section 10(7). In addition, sections 67 and 68 obligate practitioners to provide an independent advocate to enable the participation of those who may otherwise find it difficult to take part in assessments and Safeguarding Adult Review processes respectively. The Local Government Association and Directors of Adult Social Services (2019) have developed a framework to support practitioners in making decisions about their duty to carry out safeguarding adult enquiries. For further reading, see Spreadbury and Hubbard (2020) and Spreadbury and Lawson (2021). Try to spend some time familiarising yourself with this framework.

The six key principles underpinning safeguarding work

In addition to the above, practitioners are obligated to use the six key principles underpinning the safeguarding (see Table 5.2) and Making Safeguarding Personal policy incorporated in the *Care Act 2014* to guide their work.

Table 5.2 The six principles underpinning safeguarding adults

Principles	What does it mean?	What does this mean to people who use services?
Empowerment	People being supported and encouraged to make their own decisions and informed consent.	I am asked what I want as the outcomes from the safeguarding process, and these directly inform what will happen.
Prevention	It is better to take action before harm occurs.	I receive clear and simple information about what abuse is, how to recognise the signs and what I can do to seek help.
Proportionality	The least-intrusive response appropriate to the risk presented.	I am sure the professionals will work in my interest, as I see them, and they will only get involved as much as needed.
Protection	Support and representation for those in greatest need.	I get help and support to report abuse and neglect. I get help so I can take part in the safeguarding process to the extent I want.
Partnership	Local solutions through services working with their communities. Communities have a part to play in preventing, detecting and reporting neglect and abuse.	I know staff treat any personal and sensitive information in confidence, only sharing what is helpful and necessary.
Accountability	Accountability and transparency in delivering safeguarding.	I understand the role of everyone involved in my life and so do they.

Source: Taken from DHSC (2024, 14.13).

Marking Safeguarding Personal

Making Safeguarding Personal (MSP) is an England sector-led initiative that was introduced in 2012 and included in the Care and Support Statutory Guidance accompanying the *Care Act 2014* when the *Care Act* was implemented in 2015 (DHSC, 2024). MSP is built on person-centred and strengths-based perspectives and is underpinned by relational ontology. It foregrounds the collaborative involvement of people who are experiencing, or may be at risk of, abuse, neglect and harm in safeguarding enquiries. MSP requires practitioners to have conversations with the person at the centre of any safeguarding concerns to ascertain their views, wishes, aspirations and desired outcomes in terms of what would make them feel safe, free from abuse, harm and neglect. This is in order to enhance choice and control, as well as promote well-being by supporting the person to achieve resolution and recovery. Engagement in MSP and professional curiosity practice are both central to safeguarding work: these allow practitioners to truly *see* the individual, hear their narrative and understand where they are coming from in order to co-create effective safety plans and interventions that meet their needs and desired outcomes. In addition to supporting the person to meet a desired outcome, good practice requires that you review the co-created safety plans to enable you and the person at the centre of the safeguarding enquiry, family, friends and carers to co-monitor the effectiveness of the safety plans to ascertain whether the desired outcomes have been achieved in line with policy and law. The annual *Safeguarding Adults Collection* (SAC) held by NHS Digital (2024b) in England includes specific questions relating to MSP. Local authorities are required to record the number of people supported to achieve both 'desired' and 'achieved outcomes' as well as the age band of the person at the centre of the safeguarding concerns (see SG4 SAC, NHS Digital, 2024b). Engagement in MSP practice encourages you to use curiosity to identify what matters to the person when there are concerns about abuse, harm and neglect. Collaborative engagement with those experiencing or at risk of abuse, harm and neglect through MSP practice involves careful listening and empathic understanding, using age-appropriate communication tools and approaches, showing interest, not judging and not taking over decisions but rather working alongside the person and supporting them to identify what they would like to change to be safe. MSP practice is person-led, recognising that some people may require support to do so. Support may involve assisting the person to articulate what is happening as well as to lead on the co-creation and implementation of protective interventions that reduce, remove or mitigate the abuse. Advocacy support will be required to enable the views and/or best interests of those unable to do so to be included. Hafford-Letchfield et al (2021, p 1099) note that the approaches used '*should involve collaborative empowerment whereby feelings of isolation and rejection can be replaced with hope, a sense of agency and belief in personal control*'.

Why is MSP important?

Research studies reporting on adult abuse identify that most abuse takes place in intra-familial relationships. A study by Yan et al (2023) that looked at risk and protective factors relating to caregiver abuse found that most of the abuse took place in existing family relationships and at the cared-for person's home. This concurs with a cross-sectional secondary data analysis of the help-seeking behaviour of victims/survivors of older people and their family and carers who sought support through national helplines (Fraga Dominguez et al, 2022). The authors found that most victims/survivors of abuse lived in privately owned homes and the perpetrator was known to the person as a spouse/partner, son, daughter, other family member, friend or neighbour (Fraga Dominguez et al, 2022). It is also important to remember that some victims/survivors of abuse live in institutions and the perpetrator may be a practitioner or fellow resident or even a colleague, as demonstrated in enquiries into care home abuse – see, for example, the SAR of Joanna, Jon and Ben, Cawston Park (Norfolk Safeguarding Adult Board, 2021). Some victims/survivors of abuse may choose to continue to see or even live with the person who is abusing them. Similarly, those living in institutions may not want to move but importantly, in both cases, would like the abuse to stop. Adopting an MPS approach and the six principles underpinning the safeguarding become very important for ascertaining the wishes and desired outcomes of the person to whom protection is owed by ensuring that their right to live safely free from abuse, neglect and harm is respected and protected. The approach also supports you as a practitioner to build on the person's strengths rather than focusing on deficits. As discussed in Chapter 3, use of a strengths-based approach (DHSC, 2019) is one of the enablers of professional curiosity practice. Research studies examining practitioners' perspectives on the benefits of MSP reports that while MSP requires more time, investment in time reduces future referrals and complaints (Ahuja et al, 2022; Hafford-Letchfield et al, 2021). See Chapter 6 for an in-depth discussion of skills, attributes and values required for partnership collaborative engagement in MSP work.

For further reading on safeguarding adults, see the Statutory Guidance Accompanying the *Care Act 2014* (DHSC, 2024, 14.7); this is updated regularly online by the Department of Health and Social Care and provides guidance on sections 42 to 46 of the *Care Act 2014*. It covers:

- adult safeguarding – what it is and why it matters;
- abuse and neglect – understanding what they are and spotting the signs;
- reporting and responding to abuse and neglect;
- carers and adult safeguarding;
- adult safeguarding procedures;
- local authority roles and multi-agency working;
- criminal offences and adult safeguarding;
- safeguarding enquiries;
- Safeguarding Adults Boards;
- Safeguarding Adults Reviews;
- information-sharing, confidentiality and record-keeping;
- roles, responsibilities and training in local authorities, the NHS and other agencies.

Other relevant areas of law

Other relevant legislation relating to collaborative work and safeguarding adult practice at the time of writing (July 2024) included the *Mental Health Act 1983*; the *Mental Health Act 1983* Code of Practice; *Mental Health Act 2007*; the *Mental Capacity Act 2005* (MCA); the *Mental Capacity Act 2005* Code of Practice and Deprivation of Liberty Safeguards (DOLs); and the *Mental Capacity (Amendment) Act 2019* and a draft Code of Practice. It is worth mentioning that mental health legislation was undergoing reforms at the time of writing. The remainder of this section looks at the mental health legislative framework in place at the time of writing.

Mental Health Act 1983

The *Mental Health Act 1983* as amended by the *Mental Health Act 2007* (MHA) provides the legislative framework for the admission, treatment, detainment and rights of individuals who have a mental disorder and who as a result are at risk of harm to themselves or to others. It applies in both England and Wales. The *Mental Health Act 2007* covers people admitted to hospital or prison, or who are on remand, as well as those living in the community. The 1983 Act is supported by a Code of Practice; this provides guidance for practitioners by clarifying roles and responsibilities as well as the rights of those who have a mental illness, their families and carers. A White Paper on reforming the *Mental Health Act* was published in 2021 with the aim of bringing mental health services in line with modern practice and strengthening the involvement of people going through mental health challenges in decisions about their care and treatment.

Mental Capacity Act 2005

Alongside the *Mental Health Act 1983* (as amended 2007) is the *Mental Capacity Act 2005* (MCA). This provision covers those aged 16 years and over and applies to England and Wales. The *MCA 2005* is also supported by a Code of Practice. In addition, the Deprivation of Liberty Safeguards (DoLs) provide for authorised deprivation of liberty for those aged 18 years and over who lack capacity to decide on their own, to enable the person to receive care and or treatment in their best interests. DoLs apply to people living in care homes or hospitals and has been extended to cover people living in the community. The *MCA 2005* provides the legislative framework for people to make their own decisions as well as assisting those who lack capacity to do so via a best interests decision-making framework (*MCA 2005*, ss 1(5) and 4). The *MCA 2005* helps practitioners to determine whether a person has or lacks mental capacity, either temporarily or permanently, to make or take a relevant decision. Capacity is defined as *'the ability to make a decision'* (Department for Constitutional Affairs, 2007, p 41). The Act also outlines who can and should make decisions on the person's behalf if they are not able to do so themselves and allows people who do have capacity to make plans for a time when they may lack capacity in the future. You may have heard about Lasting Power of Attorney or Enduring Power of Attorney; the Act allows people to appoint an attorney to act on their behalf should they lose capacity in the future through the use of a Lasting Power of Attorney. It is not possible now to make an Enduring Power of Attorney, although if such a power was created prior to the implementation of the MCA in 2007 it is still considered to be valid once registered.

Engagement in collaborative practice requires that you involve appointed attorneys in decision-making processes if the person at the centre of the safeguarding concern cannot do so themselves. The MCA provides further provision to support those who lack capacity to make decisions for themselves through the appointment of an Independent Mental Capacity Advocate (IMCA) for those who lack capacity but have no one to speak on their behalf. In certain safeguarding situations, an IMCA might be appointed for an individual even if there are others – such as family members – who might be able to speak for them. The five statutory principles underpinning the *Mental Capacity Act 2005*, as set out in section 1(1)–(6), are as follows:

Section 1(2) A person must be assumed to have capacity unless it is established that he lacks capacity.

Section 1(3) A person is not to be treated as unable to make a decision unless all practicable steps to help him to do so have been taken without success.

Section 1(4) A person is not to be treated as unable to make a decision merely because he make an unwise decision.

Section 1(5) An act done, or decision made, under this Act for or on behalf of a person who lacks capacity must be done, or made, in his best interests.

Section 1(6) Before the act is undertaken or the decision is made, regard must be had to whether the purpose for which it is needed can be as effectively achieved in a way that is less restrictive.

Professional curiosity: capacity assessment and partnerships work

You have legal obligations to work collaboratively with those who have a mental illness and/or mental health challenges and to involve them in decision-making processes. A starting point when applying MCA 2005 is a presumption of capacity, this is fundamental to the Act. The Act stipulates that a person must be assumed to have capacity unless it is established that they lack capacity (MCA 2005, s 1(2)). In a Court of Protection judgment, *Warrington Borough Council v Y & Ors* [2023] EWCOP 27, Hayden J emphasised the importance of the presumption of capacity, noting that it *'is a powerful safeguard of civil liberty'* which *'requires to be rebutted on cogent evidence'*. This means you cannot deny justice to the person at the heart of any safeguarding concern without the evidence to support the conclusion that they do not have capacity without taking the necessary steps to establish their capacity to take or make decisions (MCA Code of Practice, 4.10). In establishing capacity, it is important to talk to the person at the centre of the safeguarding concern if there is any doubt that they may lack capacity and also to support them to take or make the decision themselves if they are able to do so. It is also important to get to know the person by finding out what is important to them and building rapport and a relationship of trust with them, as doing so will put the person at ease. Evidence from SARs indicates that building rapport and relationships of trust with those at the centre of safeguarding concerns is essential for successful engagement. For example, in the SAR of Adult H, it was reported that a judge gained Adult H's trust by engaging him in a conversation about football and by doing so learnt more about Adult H in that short conversation than other professionals who had tried for weeks to engage Adult H in matters relating to his health and immigration status (Sandiford, 2023b, 6.108).

Two components of capacity assessment: decisional capacity and executive functional capacity

Case law delineates two components of capacity: decisional capacity and executive functional capacity. Decisional capacity relates to the ability to understand and reason through the elements of the decision that needs to be made. In contrast, executive functioning is described as *'the ability to think, act, and solve problems, including the functions of the brain which help us learn new information, remember and retrieve the information we've learned in the past, and use this information to solve problems of everyday life'* (A Local Authority v AW [2020] EWCOP 24 paragraph 39). These two components are important for determining capacity. For example, some people can say they will be able to carry out a specific task, which may suggest they can do so, but at the same time they may lack the ability or motivation to convert what they say into action. Decisional capacity and executive functional capacity are important when there is a dissociation between knowing and understanding the nature of the decision and the ability to follow through on this by converting what one says into action due to an impairment in the functions of the mind. Carrying out both decisional and executive functional capacity assessments promotes curiosity by enabling practitioners to unpick whether the person can enact a decision they have made. In *Warrington Borough Council v Y & Ors* [2023] EWCOP 27, Hayden J noted that it is important *'to provide a scaffolding of support [for the people you work with] in order that [they] are availed of the very best opportunity to reassert [their] autonomy in these two very important spheres of decision taking'*. Executive functioning can be assessed by using prompt questions such as 'Tell me' and/or 'Show me'. If, having done all this, you conclude that a person has capacity to take action as well as making the decision, there is a legal obligation to record and document the rationale for assuming capacity. If, however, you are still concerned that the person may lack capacity to make a decision (even with support to do so), you are required to carry out the two-stage functional test of capacity as set out under section 2 of the *Mental Capacity Act 2005* as shown here:

> *Stage 1: Does the person have an impairment or disturbance of the mind? (Examples may include illnesses such a mental health problem, dementia, stroke, a learning disability, confusion, or drowsiness, brain injury, or alcohol misuse.) Where this exists:*
>
> *Stage 2: Is the impairment/illness causing the person to be unable to make these particular decisions?*
>
> *If capacity is in doubt, carry out the four-points capacity test.*
>
> *Section 3 (1) of MCA 2005 indicates that an individual is deemed to lack capacity if they are unable to (functional element):*
>
> - *understand the information relevant to the decision;*
> - *retain that information;*
> - *use or weigh that information as part of the process of making the decision; or*

- *communicate his decision (whether by talking, using sign language or any other means).*

Capacity assessment is time (when the issues occur) and decision (what the decision is about) specific (MCA 2005, s 2(1) and MCA Code of Practice, 2013, 4.4). For further reading, see the judicial guidance in *PC v City of York Council* 2014 2 WLR 1 and *B v A Local Authority* [2019] 3 WLR 685.

Following the decisional and executive functional assessments, if it is determined that the person has capacity, it is important to record this and to continue to support the person with the needs and outcomes that they want to achieve. You are required by law to take into account any fluctuating capacity; a key question to ask is whether the person's capacity changes frequently or a change has been brought on due to the impact of mental illness, other illness, medication or changes in medication, alcohol or drug misuse disorder or shock? In such cases, consider whether the assessment could be delayed if the person may regain capacity and the lack of capacity is of a temporary nature. However, if it is determined following the functional test that the person lacks capacity, and that they are unable to make the relevant decisions due to an impairment or disturbance in mind or brain, you are required to take action in the person's best interest under section 5 of *MCA 2005*. This can be done by appointing an Independent Mental Capacity Advocate (*MCA 2005*, ss 35–41) to act on their behalf if they do not have any friends or family members who can do this (see note about appointment and use of IMCAs in situations of safeguarding). This action interfaces with Article 8 of the *Human Rights Act 1998*, the right to private and family life, and should be done in a thoughtful way. The Court of Protection (COP), established under sections 45–47 of *MCA 2005*, has jurisdiction relating to *MCA 2005*. It is the final arbiter in matters relating to capacity decisions on issues relating to the personal welfare, healthcare, property and financial affairs of those who lack mental capacity to make decisions for themselves, and any unresolved issues should be referred to the court. For further reading on research studies that have examined disputes on mental capacity decisions presented to the Court of Protection, see Ruck Keene et al (2019). Examining these cases and the approaches used will deepen your understanding of working collaboratively, not only with the person at the centre of safeguarding concerns but also with regard to professional decision-making when using collaborative approaches and partnerships in safeguarding work.

APPLYING CONCEPTS TO PRACTICE

Scenario

Imagine that you are working at a police station and had a referral relating to T, a 41 year-old white British male. T has been assaulted and sustained a life-threatening injury, but he is refusing to seek medical help. T is known to professionals. He is the eldest of five siblings and enjoys cycling and playing football. T struggles with drug misuse and mental health challenges. He receives buprenorphine on prescription

→

98 • Professional Curiosity in Safeguarding Adults

> from a local drug and alcohol service. He was released from prison some three months ago after serving a ten-year prison sentence for assaulting his wife. It is reported that T obtained qualifications in gardening and carpentry during his time in prison. T was detained under section 2 of the *Mental Health Act* about three months ago due to deterioration in his mental health. He has a tenancy but believes he is being persecuted and therefore sleeps rough. T is known to have made repeated calls to the ambulance service and attended Accident and Emergency Services on numerous occasions relating to pain and mental health. Reports from Probation Services suggest T has difficulties with interpersonal skills, can be aggressive, uses abusive and threatening language and intercuts conversations.

TASK

- What are your initial thoughts?
- How would you use professional curiosity and law to work collaboratively with T and others?
- What are the potential challenges and how do you plan to address these?
- Now read the case on which this scenario is based (Ward, 2024).
- Make a list of what you have learnt from this case.
- How would you use what you have learnt to inform future practice?

In relation to T, the law requires that you must start from the assumption that T has capacity unless it is established that he lacks capacity (s 1(2)). Paragraph 2.4 of the MCA Code of Practice establishes that:

> *It is important to balance people's right to make a decision with their right to safety and protection when they can't make decisions to protect themselves. But the starting assumption must always be that an individual has the capacity, until there is proof that they do not.*

You might have identified, in T's case, the existence of the mental illness, alcohol use disorder and the sustained life-threatening injury (Stage 1). The next step is to establish whether the impairment/life-threatening injury is causing T to be unable to make a decision to seek medical help as required (Stage 2). It is important to remember that the law specifies that a person lacks capacity if they are unable to understand, retain or weigh up information to make the decision. In T's case, the decision to seek medical treatment at that specific time needs to be established. Partnership working and your legal obligations require that all efforts should be made to support T to make the decision (MCA

2005, s 1(3)), and if he is unable to do so you are required to consider why you were unable to assist T to take the decision. You might want to ask whether it is the right time to carry out the capacity decision assessment when he is unwell or, if it is the first time you have met T, to ask whether he would prefer to have someone he knows present while supporting him to take the decision, or whether you have provided sufficient information about different options to enable T to weigh up the different options and choose one. Good practice requires that care should be taken when giving options, in order to not unduly influence the options given: *Re ZK (No 2)* [2021] EWCOP 61 at paragraph 19; *PH v A Local Authority, Z Ltd and R* [2011] EWHC 1704 (Fam); *Oldham MBC v GW and PW* [2007] EWHC 136 (Fam). Within an assessment, you need to establish a safe space and give the person time. Where possible, an MCA assessment may need to be carried out over a period of time to give the person an opportunity to build trust. If, having taken these steps, you come to the conclusion that T lacks mental capacity to seek treatment for the life-threatening injury sustained, a medical treatment intervention decision needs to be made in his best interest.

A key question to ask is whether T will die within the next few hours if he does not receive treatment for the life-threatening injuries? If this is the case, practitioners can step in to ensure that he receives the necessary treatment. Section 5 of *MCA 2005* provides protection for such an action by allowing practitioners to implement healthcare interventions in such emergencies even if T objects. Any decisions in such cases must be proportionate and appropriate, and should be in the best interest of T. An Independent Mental Capacity Advocate should be appointed (MCA 2005, ss 35–41) to assist if T has no family or friends who could take decisions in his best interests. The case study suggests that T is the eldest of five siblings – this provides the opportunity to ask curious questions about the siblings. It is also important to use curiosity to establish how T came to sustain the injury. Is he under any coercive control? When working with someone who has experienced coercion and control, it can be difficult to establish whether they are saying what the perpetrator wants them to say or has told them say, or whether they simply cannot enact their decision. The inherent jurisdiction of the High Court may need to be considered in the cases of adults who have capacity to make decisions that may result in them placing themselves at risk of significant harm or death (*DL V a Local Authority and Others* [2012]).

Mental Capacity (Amendment) Act 2019

As mentioned previously, mental health law was undergoing reforms at the time of writing this book. The *Mental Capacity (Amendment) Act 2019* (MC(A)A) received Royal Assent on 16 May 2022. It reformed the *MCA 2005* by introducing Liberty Protection Safeguards (LPS), a new process for authorising deprivations of liberty for those who lack decision-making capacity (Garratt and Laing, 2022). LPS applies to those aged 16 years and over and living in their own home, family home, supported living, care homes and hospital. MC(A)A 2019 was meant to be implemented in October 2020 alongside LPS in April 2022. As part of this process, a 16-week public consultation on the proposed changes to a Mental Capacity Code of Practice was launched by the previous UK government in March 2022. The proposed changes included how a person's capacity to make a decision is defined and how it should be assessed under the two-stage test capacity assessment. For example, among others the draft Code of Practice stipulated that

> *an assessor should firstly consider whether the person is able to make the decision, and if not, whether there is an impairment or disturbance in the functioning of the mind or brain causing their inability to make the decision.*
>
> (HM Government, 2022 1.3, p 19)

As stated, LPS were meant to replace DoLS; however, on 5 April 2023, the Department of Health and Social Care announced that implementation of the LPS would be delayed beyond the life of the then parliament (the Sunak administration in government at that point). DoLS was still in place at the time of writing in July 2024. Following the Labour government general election victory on 4 July 2024, the new government announced its commitment to reforming mental health legislation in the King's Speech given on 17 July 2024. The Labour government's legislation plan aims to '*give patients greater choice, autonomy, enhanced rights and support, and ensure everyone is treated with dignity and respect throughout treatment*' (Labour Party, 2024, p 102). We still don't know when LPS would come into force and if it does, what shape it might take. It is very important to familiarise yourself with any new changes in law as it would have a retrospective impact on practice.

Other relevant legislation

Equivalent mental capacity legislation exists in Scotland (*Adults with Incapacity (Scotland) Act 2000*) and Northern Ireland (*Mental Capacity Act (Northern Ireland) 2016*). Other key relevant legislative frameworks embedding collaborative and partnership work in safeguarding work include the *Health and Care Act 2022* (this provides the legislative framework for integration of services between health and social care), the *Human Rights Act 1998* (Art 2 right to life; Art 3 no torture, inhuman or degrading treatment; Art 4 freedom from slavery and forced labour; Art 5 liberty and security; Art 6 right to a fair trial; and Art 8 right to respect for a private and family life), the *Equality Act 2010* (s 4 protected characteristics and s 20 duty to make reasonable adjustments), the *Domestic Abuse Act 2021* and the *Data Protection Act 2018*. For more reading from the series see Starns (2019) and Feldon (2024), which both provide a comprehensive coverage of the legislative context of safeguarding adults.

Legislative context of work in the other three nations of the United Kingdom

Wales

In Wales, alongside the *MHA 1983, MCA 2005* and *MA(A)A 2019* and their accompanying Codes of Practice, the main legislative framework for safeguarding adult exists in the

Social Services and Wellbeing (Wales) Act 2014. This applies to individuals aged 18 years and over who are experiencing or are at risk of abuse and neglect, and have needs for care and support (whether or not the authority is meeting any of those needs), and as a result of those needs cannot protect themselves against abuse or neglect. Other relevant law includes the *Violence Against Women, Domestic Abuse and Sexual Violence (Wales) Act 2015* and the National Wales Safeguarding Procedures (2021), the *Equality Act 2010* and the *Human Rights Act 1998*.

Northern Ireland

There is no one single legislative framework that guides safeguarding adults practice in Northern Ireland. Safeguarding adult legislation is set out under the *Domestic Abuse and Civil Proceedings Act (Northern Ireland) 2021*, Safeguarding Vulnerable Groups (NI) Order 2007, the *Criminal Law Act (NI) 1967* and the *Human Rights Act 1998*. The Department of Health (2021) in Northern Ireland held an open consultation on legislative options to develop an Adult Protection Bill but no legislation has resulted from this to date.

Scotland

In Scotland, the governing legislation for safeguarding adults is the *Adult Support and Protection (Scotland) Act 2007*. This creates a legal framework for local authorities in Scotland to protect adults from harm and abuse, including self-harm. The legislation is supported by the Adult Support and Protection Improvement Plan 2019–22 (Scottish Government, 2019). Inter-agency and interdisciplinary cooperation are enshrined under section 5 of the *Adult Support and Protection (Scotland) Act 2007*. An 'adult at risk' of harm, abuse and neglect is defined under Section 3(1) as those who are:

- unable to safeguard their own well-being, property, rights or other interests;
- at risk of harm; and
- because they are affected by disability, mental disorder, illness or physical or mental infirmity, more vulnerable to being harmed than adults who are not so affected.

And under Section 3(2) where:

- another person's conduct is causing (or likely to cause) the adult to be harmed; or
- the adult is engaging (or likely to engage) in conduct which causes (or is likely to cause) self-harm.

Table 5.3 provides a summary of the main UK legislative framework for safeguarding adults that you might find useful.

Table 5.3 Summary of the main UK legislative framework for safeguarding adults

Four nations of the United Kingdom	Safeguarding adult legislation	Mental capacity law
England	The Care Act 2014	Mental Capacity Act 2005; Mental Capacity (Amendment) Act 2019
Wales	Social Services and Wellbeing (Wales) Act 2014	Mental Capacity Act 2005; Mental Capacity (Amended) Act 2019
Northern Ireland	Adult Safeguarding Prevention and Protection in Partnership, 2015 (DHSSPS and DoJ, 2015)	Mental Health (Northern Ireland) Order 1986; Mental Capacity Act (Northern Ireland) 2016
Scotland	Adult Support and Protection (Scotland) Act 2007	Adult with Incapacity (Scotland) Act 2000
Human Rights Act 1998 Equality Act 2010 (except Northern Ireland – only some sections apply		

International comparisons

Like the United Kingdom, New Zealand has a statutory (functional) mental capacity test assessment under its *Personal and Property Rights Act 1998* (PPPR Act); this is applied by judges of the Family Court and High Court (Douglass, 2016; Ruck Keene et al, 2019). Davidson et al (2024) report that, like the four nations of the United Kingdom, Australia, Canada, Finland, France, Germany, New Zealand, Norway and Sweden all emphasise the importance of using co-production approaches to identify what is important to those at the centre of safeguarding concerns when determining mental capacity. The authors also reported that, similar to the four nations of the United Kingdom, data about the use of mental health and mental capacity laws in the aforementioned countries tend to focus on activities and processes rather than on exploration of the people's experiences about the processes (Davidson et al, 2024). This highlights the importance of seeking as well as using feedback from people who use services as part of collaborative approaches to improve practice.

KEY POINTS FROM THIS CHAPTER

- Partnership work achieved through collaborative practice and joined-up working with professionals and people at the centre of safeguarding concerns are central to professional curiosity practice and safeguarding work.

- Working in partnership with people at the centre of safeguarding enquiries requires their involvement in decisions about what needs to be done to make them feel safe and their involvement in co-creating interventions that keep their desired and achieved outcomes at the centre. These are central to MSP practice.

- Ask curious questions about how things appear, how things are done within multi-professional inter-agency contexts where challenges exist in relationships with others, in teams and with the people with whom you are working. Use self and perspective talking to explore and understand as well as challenge inappropriate practice.

- The legal and policy frameworks in safeguarding work are complex and need carefully consideration to ensure rights to protection are respected.

- You are uniquely placed to use the legal mandate invested in you to ensure that the rights of those experiencing abuse, harm and neglect and their families are respected and protected.

Further reading

B v A Local Authority [2019] 3 WLR 685
Provides judicial guidance on making decision and time specific capacity assessment.

PC v City of York Council [2014] 2 WLR 1
Provides judicial guidance on making decisions.

Ruck Keene, A, Kane, N B, Kim, S Y H and Owen, G S (2019) Taking Capacity Seriously? Ten Years of Mental Capacity Disputes Before England's Court of Protection. *International Journal of Law Psychiatry*, 62: 56–76. https://doi.org/10.1016/j.ijlp.2018.11.005.
Provides some examples of cases that have come before the Court of Protection.

6 Putting partnership work into practice

> **CHAPTER OBJECTIVES**
>
> By the end of this chapter, you should be able to:
>
> - know the core skills that underpin professionally curious and partnership work;
> - demonstrate knowledge and skills for collaborative working with those at the centre of safeguarding enquiries when engaging in professional curiosity practice;
> - demonstrate knowledge and skills for collaborative working with other professionals involved in safeguarding enquiries;
> - harness the opportunities of using digital technology to connect with others.

Introduction

Earlier chapters in this book have considered skills required more generally for professional curiosity practice. This chapter further examines the core skills, attributes and values underpinning professional curiosity and partnership work with those owed a duty of care and protection from abuse, neglect and harm, and their families and carers. The discussions include the skills required for partnership work with other professionals in multi-agency and interdisciplinary work at both frontline and managerial levels. The chapter concludes by suggesting some new ways of working in a post-pandemic world and how to harness the opportunities of using digital technology to connect with others, including practice implications. Case examples and learning are drawn from SARs, enabling you to think through the skills and attributes required for effective engagement in collaborative partnership with those at the centre of safeguarding enquiries, families, carers and colleagues (other professionals). The chapter begins by considering the core skills underpinning professional curiosity and partnership with those at risk of abuse, harm and neglect.

Core skills underpinning professional curiosity and partnership with service users

Communication and the ability to build trust are central to collaborative partnership work with those at the centre of safeguarding enquiries. Core skills required include empathy, compassion, co-identification of risk, negotiation, liaising and co-creation of interventions that supports the individual, their families and carers. Underpinning all these skills (aforementioned) is active listening and understanding. As you might have gathered from Chapter 5, the policies and legal frameworks that guide safeguarding practice are procedural and process driven. However, engagement in professional curiosity practice and partnership work requires that you go beyond the procedural process-driven practice by getting to know people.

First and foremost, engagement in partnership work with those at the centre of safeguarding concerns centres on seeing and valuing the person as an individual human being, worthy and deserving of your time, attention and interest. You do so by spending time to understand the person – what they might be going through, including relevant risks, strengths, capabilities, fears, anxieties; what might be informing or framing their decisions and choices – and gaining and building a relationship of trust with them. Your practice and engagement should enable those at the centre of safeguarding concerns to *'feel seen, heard and valued'* (Vogel and Flint 2021, p 35). This may involve listening and listening again, using cultural curiosity, perspective-taking, critical thinking and analysis, critical reflection, negotiation, judgement and decision-making. This may require the use of appropriate frameworks to understand what they may be going through and providing the resources to support them. Abuse, harm and neglect encompass physical, psychological and emotional pain and suffering. They also involve social shame, which means it can be challenging for some people to open up while others may not have the concepts to explain what they are going through, and still others might perceive what they are going through as not unusual because they might not have known any other way. It is important to remember that you are well placed as a practitioner to know, understand and work 'with' people to support them. What follows looks at the concept of empathy and the skill required for engagement in empathic practice with people who are at risk of or experiencing abuse, neglect and harm.

The concept of empathy

The concept of empathy is complex and multifaceted. There is no one agreed definition of what is meant by empathy (Cuff et al, 2016; Delgado et al, 2023). Empathy is associated with perspective-taking, emotion sharing and compassion. Burnard (1992, p 69) defines empathy as *'the ability to enter the perceptual world of the other person: to see the world as they see it. It also suggests an ability to cover this identification of feelings to the other person'*. Studies examining the concept of empathy suggest it is something that we 'think' (cognitive), 'feel' (affective) and 'do' (behaviour) (King, 2011; Riess, 2017). The domains of 'thinking' (cognitive), 'feeling' (affective) and 'doing' (behaviour) are interdependent and seen as processes. The cognitive domain includes perspective-taking and interpersonal sensitivity, while the affective domain involves caring and congruence. The behavioural domain covers selflessness and therapeutic relationship (King, 2011). Delgado et al (2023) note that empathy helps us to connect by *feeling* with others. For example, affective empathy involves empathic concerns and personal distress, which are expressed through the ability to recognise others' distress and respond with compassion, thoughtfulness and care. Efilti and Gelmez (2023, p 122) note that empathy *'requires a skilful activity that is the expansion of one's consciousness by including the other'*. Concurring with King (2011) and Riess (2017), Depow et al (2021, p 1199) note that *'empathy allows us to connect with other people by taking their perspective, sharing their emotions, and feeling compassion for them'*. Empathy is viewed as a personality trait, capabilities, skills and attitudes that can be learnt (Riess, 2017). Empathy is underpinned by relational ontology and is essential in human relational connectedness. Research studies that have examined the concept of empathy indicate that empathy is experienced through understanding, sharing emotion and compassion (Depow et al, 2021).

Interpersonal empathic skills are therefore essential in collaborative partnership work with people who are experiencing or at risk of abuse, harm and neglect. It helps practitioners to anticipate and understand their emotions as well as the emotional state of others and their behaviour to modify their decisions and actions accordingly. Empathy also involves the ability to work towards a shared goal; it is useful both when working with people who use services and when working with colleagues in inter-agency/multidisciplinary or interprofessional practice. Weisz and Cikara (2021, p 213) point out that empathy allows us in this context to *'cultivate and transmit knowledge, and to coordinate collective action toward shared goals'*. Safeguarding work is complex, and it may not always be possible for all to agree on what it means to be safe and how to mitigate perceived and identified risk, as discussed in Chapter 4. Perspective-taking is a key component of empathy, central to listening and understanding the perspectives of others from their point of view. Perspective-taking is the *process* by which people take the perspective of others (when we imagine another person's point of view) and work with them from their point of view. Citing Ku et al (2015), Calvard et al (2023, p 35) note that perspective-taking relates to: *'the active cognitive process of imagining the world from another's vantage point or imagining oneself in another's shoes to understand their visual viewpoint, thoughts, motivations, intentions, and/or emotions'*.

Perspective-taking is crucially important for understanding how those at the centre of safeguarding enquiries perceive the risk of harm, abuse and neglect, and what they wish to change and/or how they want to see that change happen. This may include, for example, helping the person to articulate what is happening to them if they are unable to do so, providing appropriate support through advocacy to enable them to recover from the abuse or supporting them by providing protective interventions that reduce or mitigate the abuse. Perspective-taking also involves the ability to attune to what others may be going through at a cognitive level rather than at an emotional level – it is goal directed. As mentioned, collaborative working involves working not only with other practitioners, but also with the person at the centre of the enquiry's family, carers and friends. This requires practitioners to listen and understand the perspectives of families, carers and friends about how risk and risk-enablement plans are conceptualised from all parties. Relationship-building and trust are therefore central to perspective-taking, as without these you will not be able to work towards a shared goal.

Involvement of people who use services in safeguarding work

Involvement of people with lived experiences in the training and education of social work students, GP training, nursing and midwifery is well established in the United Kingdom and internationally (Anka and Taylor, 2016; Stanley and Webber, 2022). Evidence suggests that service user involvement has positive impacts on students. The inclusion of family perspectives in SARs provides insights about the impact of how professionals worked with them and how they would have liked professionals to have worked with them. In the SAR concerning Harry, the author notes:

> Harry's parents had strong feelings about Harry's mental capacity, and what this meant for his life. Harry's mum said, "Whenever it was quoted, I would want to scream." It was her "most hated word with so many meanings". It would either be an excuse to discharge Harry from a service, or a reason to make him do something that he did not want to do. From her perspective mental capacity was at the centre of everything, but never anything positive for Harry.
>
> (Barnsley Safeguarding Adult Board, 2023, p 20, 6.6.3)

A starting point to learn how to collaborate in partnership with those at the centre of safeguarding enquiries and their families is involving them in risk-identification and risk-enablement assessments, as well as developing risk plans that are co-produced. Involvement should extend beyond frontline practice to a more strategic level in planning and commissioning of services to enable practitioners to develop deeper relationships of trust by learning with and from people with lived experiences. Muirden and Appleton's (2022) integrative review of the literature focusing on how health and social care practitioners exercised professional curiosity in child protection practice found relationship-building between practitioners and people using services influenced in-depth information elicitation between practitioners and those using services. Of the 1428 papers reviewed, which focused on papers published between 2000 and 2019, 24 studies met their inclusion criteria. Other relevant skills required for engaging in collaborative partnership work with those at risk of and/or experiencing abuse, harm and neglect include critical thinking and analysis, negotiations and the ability to liaise.

Critical thinking and analysis

Like the concept of empathy, the concept of critical thinking is difficult to define as different disciplines define it differently. Rawles (2023, p 115) notes that critical thinking involves *'being skeptical and questioning everything that you read, see or hear, then analysing and evaluating it before drawing conclusion'*. In simple terms, critical thinking involves the ability to examine, explore, reflect and evaluate things in more depth. It involves the ability to examine things from different perspectives, weigh up different options and objectives, and use different knowledge types to evaluate and examine the information gathered to make informed judgements about decisions made. Key skills used in critical thinking include logical thinking and judgement formulation, evaluation, synthesis, reasoning, problem-solving, intuition, imagination and creativity (Santos Meneses, 2020). Boryczko (2022) notes that critical thinking provides the opportunity to address gaps in cumulative knowledge, which aligns with the four types of curious people discussed in Chapter 1.

In safeguarding work, engagement in critical thinking may involve, for example, undertaking critical incident analysis and examining and evaluating contextual factors and background information, including analysis of socio-structural determinants and how these affect the person. Such determinants include age, disabilities, gender, race, religion and sexuality, as well as socio-economic and political factors. Critical thinking and analysis also include the ability to examine intersectional factors to discern oppression, issues of power, epistemic injustice and human rights-related factors in the context of safeguarding and partnership work. Critical thinking in this sense calls for action, which includes *'identification and challenging assumptions'* (Brookfield, 1997, pp 7–9).

Earlier writers viewed critical thinking as constituted of cognitive, emotional attitude, ethical and sociopolitical dimensions. More recently, writers such as Santos Meneses (2020) and Boryczko (2022) have argued for a rethinking of the concept to one that is more inclusive and balances skills and dispositions with civic, ethical and cultural sensitivity. Drawing from some of the key writers in the field, these authors argue that a skills-based conception of critical thinking is less focused on morality and/or ethical values and morality (Santos Meneses, 2020; Boryczko, 2022). One example is consideration of how context might impact practice (the ability to engage in critical thinking and analysis) and the need to use supervision to discuss matters and seek help. For more reading on critical thinking, including the theories underpinning it, see Santos Meneses (2020) and Rawles (2023).

APPLYING CONCEPTS TO PRACTICE
Case study

G is in his late seventies and lives alone in rented accommodation. G has health and social care needs and requires both medical and social care support to manage these. G is a very private person and has expressed that he does not like people intruding into his life.

> Imagine that you are working at a GP surgery; you have tried on several occasions to contact G for appointment visits and have been unsuccessful. You have now referred G to social services and understand from discussions with colleagues that a practitioner has been allocated to work with G but they have also not been successful in contacting him.

TASK

- What are your initial thoughts?
- How would you use the concept of empathy and critical thinking and analysis to inform your work with G?
- Now read the case on which this scenario is based (Robson, 2024) and consider your initial thoughts, your proposed approach and what you would like to do differently.
- Make a list of what you have learnt from this case.
- How would you use what you have learnt to inform future practice?
- Use supervision to discuss the emotional impact this case may have had on you.

As mentioned in this chapter, critical thinking calls for action. Following this, the chapter now looks at the concept of compassion, which is our emotional response to empathy.

The concept of compassion

The literature tells us that *'our capacity to perceive and resonate with others' suffering allows us to feel and understand their pain'* (Resis, 2017, p 75). Compassion is concerned with the suffering of both self and others, and with taking actions to alleviate this suffering. The literature delineates two components of compassion: affective (also referred to as emotional) and behavioural. The affective component activates the emotional responses when you witness the suffering of others, which then cultivates the behavioural component – the desire to act to relieve the suffering. Strauss et al (2016) note that compassion involves the ability to recognise suffering, show understanding of the universality of human suffering, feel for the person suffering, tolerate uncomfortable feelings and be motivated to act to mitigate suffering. This is corroborated by Gilbert (2013), who notes that compassion centres on *'basic kindness, with a deep awareness of the suffering of oneself and of other living things, coupled with the wish and effort to relieve it'*. Singer and Klimeck (2014, p R875) also note that compassion is associated with the *'feelings of warm, concern and care for the other, it is a strong motivation to improve the other's wellbeing'*. Characterised by care for the well-being of others, Tanner (2020) suggests compassion does not seek to change the individual but rather seeks to work with the individual to alleviate the suffering.

Compassion and partnership work with people using services is embedded in a number of professional codes of conduct – for example, those used in nursing and midwifery (Nursing and Midwifery Council, 2018), social work (BASW, 2014) and also within NHS strategic plans (NHS England 2023a, 2023b) While much has been written about the concept of compassion in nursing, Tanner (2020) notes that little attention has been given to the concept in the social work literature. Although it is highly valued by people using social work services, it has also been found to be lacking in provision of social work services. Alongside other, interpersonal qualities and attributes such as empathy, critical thinking and analysis, compassion is noted as good practice in analysis of SARs (Preston-Shoot et al, 2024). Compassion is cited as important for effective collaborative partnership work with those at the centre of safeguarding. It foregrounds relationship-building and seeks to understand the intricate circumstances that positioned the person at the centre of a safeguarding enquiry in the position they are in. Cultivating and building positive relationships with people are central to that effect. This makes the ability and skill to build relationships of trust with the individual an important first step. Anstiss et al (2020) propose six action points that can help practitioners develop competence in using compassion. These involve being self-aware and sensitive to your own emotions and body state, being courageous and skilful in using helpful scenarios and problem-solving skills (Anstiss et al, 2020). Other core skills include being sensitive to others' distress, being moved to do something to alleviate the distress, being tolerant towards your own personal distress and being non-judgemental (Anstiss et al, 2020; Poorkavoos 2016; Vogel and Flint, 2021). Drawing from the Compassion in the Workplace model developed by the Roffey Park Institute, Vogel and Flint (2021) point out that the first step of developing competence in compassion involves being sensitive about the well-being of others. Alongside using empathy, critical thinking and analysis and compassion, what follows looks at probing, a useful communication technique that can support you to develop competence in working with others in a thoughtful partnership and a collaborative way.

Probes

Probing is a useful communication skill when engaging in professional curiosity and safeguarding practice. However, insufficient probing and analysis have been linked to a lack of professional curiosity in enquiries into the serious harm or death of adults and children. References to insufficient probing and analysis were cited in a SAR commissioned by Leeds Safeguarding Adults Board Safeguarding Adults Review of Mr A and Mrs A (Braye and Preston-Shoot, 2020) and the West Sussex Safeguarding Adults Board Safeguarding Adults Review in respect of MS (Simmons, 2019). Further, a search on the SAR national database at the end of June 2024 using the search term *'insufficient probing'* yielded 240 SARs where a lack of sufficient probing was mentioned as a factor in the serious harm or death of the adult. This highlights the importance of using probes in partnership collaboration enquiries with people in safeguarding work. Probes can be both verbal and non-verbal. They are used to explore, investigate or examine information or events in more depth.

Probes allow practitioners to seek further information to previously answered or unanswered questions. Probing is used in counselling, social work, the criminal justice system, nursing and midwifery, as well as other health and care professions. Probing underscores the concept of recognition that we are not making assumptions or judgements about a person's way of life or what is happening to them without finding out information from them or those around them in a compassionate way to establish what might be happening and what support might be appropriate. Egan (2018) points out that probes enable people to know that you are with them to encourage them to talk further.

A different taxonomy of probe types has been developed for research interview exchange that could be applied in safeguarding enquiries. Most of the theoretical frameworks underpinning the use of probes have been developed either from the field of counselling or from qualitative research. Gorden (1987) delineates six types of probes. These are: silent probe, encouragement probe, elaboration probe, clarifying probe, recapitalisation probe and reflective probe. Bernard (2013) built on Gorden's work by developing seven types of probes. Bernard's and Gorden's taxonomies of probe types overlap. For example, Bernard's taxonomy of probe types also consists of silence probe, echo probe, affirmation probe (uh-huh), which is similar to Gorden's encouragement probe and the tell-me-more probe (also similar to Gorden's encouragement probe or elaboration probe). Bernard's other probes are long probe, leading (directive) probe and baiting probe.

More recently, drawing from these earlier works, Robinson (2023) has developed a new taxonomy of probe types called the DICE approach to probing (which can also be used in research interviews). DICE stands for descriptive, idiographic, clarifying and explanatory probes. The DICE model is underpinned by narrative theory, which views narrative as co-constructed by the teller and the listener, autobiographical memory theory, self-disclosure theory and attribution theory. The DICE model is useful for examining both external events and actions, as well as internal subjective experiences – or what Robinson (2023, p 385) refers to as *'the inner landscape of consciousness'.*

When used compassionately and sensitively, probes can help you find out more about what is going on in a person's life, both externally (physically) and internally (emotionally) in conversation with others. In safeguarding work, probes can be used for identification and analysis of risk, capabilities, strengths and assets. Probes can equally be used to explore as well as co-create risk-enablement plans with those at the centre of safeguarding enquiries, with families and with other professionals. Robinson (2023) notes that external descriptive probes can be used to explore external factors such as when an event occurred – phrases such as *'when did it occur, what were you doing at the time, or what was X doing at the time'* could be used. Contextual external probes can also be used to explore contextual factors that impinge on an event. Helpful phrases drawn from Robinson (2023, p 385) include: *'What else was going on in your life at the time or what was happening in the run up to the event?'* Extension or nudging probes are also useful for facilitating the development of discussions when trying to fill in information or knowledge gap. Examples include: *'Tell me about what happened next'*; *'Is there anything that you could remember?'*; *'What sort of impact do you think X would have on Z or the whole family/team?'* Time-specific probes are used for establishing temporary factors; an example of a question that could be asked is: *'Could you give me an example of when …?'*

Explanatory probes can also be used to explore why a particular event or incident occurred. Some helpful questions drawn from Robinson (2023, p 388) include: *'Why do you personally think x happened?'* or *'What do you feel were the reasons for x occurring or in your view, what were the causes that led to x?'*. Similarly, clarification or exemplification probes could be used to enable you to understand more clearly what is going on in the person's life when this is unclear, or where you are unsure. Examples include situations where the person tells you they are fine, good or worried. Here, internal description probes that focus on subjective emotions, thoughts and feelings could be used to explore the subjective internal feelings of the person. In this context, probes such as these could be used: *'Can you explain or describe to me what fine means or what does fine or good look like?'* or *'What would have to change in order for x to happen?'* Consensus probes are useful when working with families or groups. These could be used to gauge group consensus. Examples might include: *'Is there anyone not happy with that?'* or *'Is everyone happy with that?'* or *'What would the family/team like to see for change to happen?'*

Equally important are clearinghouse probes, these allow the person at the centre of safeguarding concerns to share with you what is on their mind that you have not previously covered (Hargie, 2016). Clearinghouse probes are important for engagement in professional curiosity practice and should be undertaken with sensitivity, thoughtfulness and kindness. Example questions such as this could be asked: *'Is there anything that I haven't asked you that is on your mind, which you would like to have been asked?'* (Hargie, 2016, p 142). Such questions would enable the person to share their perspectives on what had happened to them. This is crucially important as practitioners/organisations may have their own agenda and can be influenced and constrained by resources; they therefore may not ask questions that are important to the person at the centre of safeguarding enquiries or their family.

You learnt from Chapter 5 that engagement in professional curiosity and partnership work with people using services require that you give voice to those experiencing harm, abuse and neglect. SARs indicate that this does not always occur. In one local child safeguarding practice review relating to Child F, commissioned by Dudley Safeguarding People Partnership and undertaken by Botham (2024), Child F's mother recounts a period in her life where she lost considerable weight due to taking illicit drugs. She described that she wanted the practitioners involved in her son's case to have shown interest in what was going on in her life by enquiring about the weight loss, but none of them did. She notes that the focus of practitioners' interactions was on her son and her use of mental health services rather than on showing additional interest in her as a person.

REFLECTIVE QUESTIONS

- Take some time to reflect on what professional curiosity and partnership work with Child F and her mother might have meant, and how you could work in partnership with both mother and child.
- What would you take forward from what Child F's mother has said to inform your own practice?

- How would you use probes to work with the family as a whole?
- Identify two resource implications that this case raises for you, which you would bring to your manager's attention.

APPLYING CONCEPTS PRACTICE
Case study

Imagine that you are working at your base team and have received a referral relating to Ms A. The referral notes suggest A is a 51-year-old, white, British woman. She lives with three generations of her family. A is reported to have several physical conditions; she is confined to her room and has not been able to leave the family home for several months. A's family is known to social services and other healthcare professionals. It is reported that A could be vulnerable to cuckooing as controlled drugs were being supplied from her home. The referral indicates that A finds it difficult to engage with services. Your team was recently called to Ms A's house and found her to be in a severely malnourished state, covered in dirt and insect bites; she also had head lice.

TASK
- How would you use the concepts of compassion and empathy to work with Ms A?
- How would you use probes to engage with Ms A and her family?
- Now read the case on which this scenario is based: see Northamptonshire Safeguarding Adults Board (2023).
- How would you use the learning from this case to inform your future practice?
- Identify three things that you would like to discuss in your team to inform good practice.
- Make a list of some of the key aspects of the case that would challenge you to use and identify one training opportunity to help you.

The involvement of other professionals in safeguarding adult work

'Think person', 'think family', 'think collaboratively'

Vogel and Flint (2021) note that we all have a natural tendency to judge others but we all also need support in tackling dilemmas that we face. It is important to 'think person' as well as 'think family' by considering the impact of the individual with care and support needs, including any safeguarding concerns, on the person at the centre of the safeguarding concerns and on the whole family. It is equally important to 'think collaboratively' and to harness support from any other professionals known to the person on how best to work together to support the person and their family. The SAR on Adult A tells us that children's services were involved with other members of the family, but practitioners worked in silos rather than together. Partnership working requires practitioners from different services involved with different members of a family to work together, taking a whole-family approach to identify need, risk of harm, abuse and neglect to provide appropriate coordinated support. Taking a 'think family' approach is emphasised in law and highlighted in the learning from the SAR of Adult A. In the SAR of Adult A, the author stressed the need for professionals to

> *consider safeguarding in its widest sense and in respect of both adults and children, recognising that whilst their individual role may relate to one aspect of the family, they also need to be alert to each family member to recognise whether there is potential evidence of abuse or apparent neglect and to take appropriate action.*
>
> (Northamptonshire Safeguarding Adults Board, 2023, p 3)

Inter-agency collaboration

The COVID-19 pandemic saw health, social care and community-based organisations coming together to find creative solutions to support those at risk of harm and abuse. To give one example, in the United Kingdom, fire and rescue services worked collaboratively with the NHS across England and Wales to support adults at risk of harm (Waring and Jones, 2023). Such collaborative partnership work included the fire and rescue services driving people to and from outpatient appointments and urgent care consultations. Good collaborative work between agencies with responsibilities to safeguard adults is central to safeguarding work and, as seen in Chapter 5, it is enshrined in law. You also learnt in Chapter 5 that some of the key components of collaboration work with other practitioners include effective communication and information-sharing, trust, respect, accountability and responsibility. Although these are important for effective inter-agency partnership and collaborative work in safeguarding work and central to professional curiosity practice, a lack of coordination and poor inter-agency work continue to be cited in reviews relating to the serious harm and deaths of children and adults. The second national analysis of SARs in England identified both shortcomings and good practice in inter-agency work (Preston-Shoot et al, 2024). Among others, these centred on poor information-sharing, an absence of case coordination, poor inter-agency referrals, failure to use inter-agency meetings and misunderstanding of data protection rules. Other shortcomings identified included a lack of multi-agency risk-management meetings and poor recordings. The authors noted:

> *Factors such as poor case coordination and information-sharing, pressures on staffing and workloads, availability of commissioned resources, and absences of*

management scrutiny, training and guidance, compromised the effectiveness of safeguarding. They have a direct influence on how practitioners in any one agency approach their work with an individual. Practitioners' awareness of these systemic factors can assist them to take appropriate actions, for example, to contribute actively to interagency coordination and information-sharing, and to escalate difficulties to the appropriate level in the safeguarding system.

(Preston-Shoot et al, 2024, p 2)

Vogel and Flint (2021, p 35) point out that '*a compassionate approach towards those experiencing moral, ethical or personal distress is essential to protect the ... workforce*'.

It is worth noting that good inter-agency practices were also identified in about a fifth of the SARs analysed (Preston-Shoot et al, 2024). The authors reported that the most commonly noted good practice centred on assessing and managing risk (this constituted 31 per cent of the cases reviewed); application of Making Safeguarding Personal principles (31 per cent of the cases); recognition of abuse and neglect, including self-neglect and continuity of involvement, and recognition and attention of health needs (each around 22 per cent) (Preston-Shoot et al, 2024). Practitioners and their managers could draw from these to inform effective inter-agency work. As with the first national analysis of SARs in England (Preston-Shoot et al, 2020), the second national analysis indicates that effective case coordination and information-sharing could be achieved by having clear protocols for how information would be shared with other professionals and agencies involved in supporting those at the centre of a safeguarding enquiry, their families and carers. In addition, multi-agency strategy meetings could be used to discuss risk and risk-management strategies, including specialist resources and expertise needed to mitigate, minimise and prevent escalation of risk. Both the national SAR analyses recommend continuing learning development of staff as well as to ensure that the resources needed are available to support the workforce. Now consider the following information from a SAR.

APPLYING CONCEPTS TO PRACTICE

Case study: learning from the SAR of Keith

Keith was a 63 year-old, white, British man. He died in hospital in 2021. Keith had health and social care needs and received services from several agencies. Keith objected to professional involvement in his life. A SAR report commissioned by Manchester Safeguarding Partnership undertaken by Ward (2023) following Keith's death suggests the core challenge of work relating to Keith centred around professional engagement, particularly around his structured programme of care. Ward (2023) notes that professionals involved in Keith's care were aware of his needs and tried to help him within their different disciplines but were unsuccessful. To give some examples, Keith declined to attend various appointments with the different practitioners involved in his care. The SAR report indicates that between October and September 2019, practitioners failed three times in their attempt to engage him to access support. In April 2020 alone, it was reported that adult social care failed in its attempt to carry out four reviews with Keith by phone and this persisted until 2021. The report provides a chronology of the attempts made and challenges encountered from 2019 to 2021. A number of serious risks were identified, including failing to attend medical treatment (failing to see a GP, declined full pressure area checks appointment, not attending outpatient respiratory appointments multiple times) and not eating and refusing support from carers.

TASK

- Work with a colleague and make a risk plan of how you might work with other agencies to support those with similar challenges to those experienced by Keith.
- Review how your organisation works with people using services, make a list of some of the current structured programmes of care in your team or approaches to practice that might not work for people in similar situations to that of Keith.
- Consider how you would bring this to the attention of your manager or team.
- Read Keith's SAR (Ward, 2023), identify one good practice in interagency collaboration and share this with your team.

Learning from the SAR of Keith: effective skills for inter-agency collaboration

In the SAR of Keith, effective referral to other agencies for support was noted as good practice; this related to a referral made to the fire service for a home safety check (Ward, 2023). Among others, Ward (2023) recommended that agencies could collaboratively work with those described as 'non-engaging' by having clear leadership, including a care coordinator and multi-agency management lead to guide the work. Ward (2023) also recommended that agencies consider appointing a multi-agency management group with responsibilities to guide, direct and support the team around the adult at the centre of safeguarding enquiry. Other recommendations included allocating a set time to complete tasks and a multi-agency team willing to be consistent and persistent. Agencies are also encouraged to have in place clear policies and procedures about how to work with those whose behaviour challenges us – those often described as 'non-engaged' or 'hard to engage'. Ward's (2023) recommendations in this area corroborate the findings from the second national analysis of SARs (Preston-Shoot et al, 2024). As well as frontline practitioners, collective agencies can collaborate by implementing risk-management plans that support those at the centre of safeguarding enquiries. Keith was said to have got on very well with his carers. Risk plans could draw from learning from the carers in relation to the approaches used that enabled them to work with Keith. Effective collaboration and partnership with people using services includes involving them in co-creating risk-enablement plans that support their needs, particularly regarding how they would like to feel safe. What follows looks at how to harness digital technology to improve collaborative partnerships.

Professional curiosity: using digital technology to connect with others

The COVID-19 pandemic gave rise to the use of digital technology to connect with others (Anka et al, 2020; Turner and Fanner, 2022). Research suggests that since the pandemic there has been an increase in text-based communication between practitioners, managers, supervisors and families (Behan-Devlin, 2024; Jeyasingham and Devlin, 2024). The literature tells us that practitioners are using mobile devices to remind people to take their medications, and also about upcoming appointments. Devices such as eye-gaze and touchscreen apps (eg Talking Matt in dementia care and learning disabilities) are used to aid communication between practitioners and people using services. Research suggests that tools such as WhatsApp have allowed young people to initiate communication with practitioners (Jeyasingham and Devlin, 2024). It is also now more common to use video-conference platforms, text or photo-messaging to connect with people. GPs now offer both telephone and video appointments. Data collected by NHS Digital (2024a) on the mode of GP appointments made in England from 1 November 2021 to 30 April 2024 suggests that there were 7,862,716 telephone GP appointments and 1,301,924 online video GP appointments made during that period.

Within the legal sphere, the Court of Protection now conducts most court proceedings online via digital platforms (see the Open Justice Court of Protection Project). In social care, research demonstrates that use of online video conferencing facilitated improved attendance at formal inter-agency/interdisciplinary meetings (eg schools, social work, GPs) (Baginsky and Manthorpe, 2021). Studies also suggest that digital technology makes practitioners more accessible to people using services. Further, studies examining social workers' digitally mediated interactions with families and other professionals suggest that judgements and professional decisions are made during these interactions. Alongside these, electronic information systems are now in place and allow different agencies and disciplines such as the NHS, social work, housing, fire services and police to share information effectively between them. In England, the Multi-Agency Safeguarding Trackers (MAST) developed by Policy in Practice (2023) allows practitioners to check whether other safeguarding agencies are actively involved with an individual, families or an address. This creates opportunities for those who are newly qualified and those in training to develop skills in using professional curiosity in these forums and/or platforms.

However, the literature in this area suggests that for those who are less experienced, this can be rather daunting. Jeyasingham and Devlin's (2024) ethnographic study with practitioners and users of children's safeguarding services in three local authorities in England draws attention to the importance of attentiveness in online virtual meetings. The researchers found that *'even when participants appeared attentive, meetings were often characterised by a flatness of emotional engagement, influencing the process of such meetings'* (Jeyasingham and Devlin, 2024, p 10). They warn that these factors, among others, can *'impede "collective intelligence" – the ability of groups to collaborate and solve problems'* (Jeyasingham and Devlin, 2024, p 10). Further, earlier research studies demonstrated that practitioners viewed digital usage as hindering practitioner relationships with people using services or were seen as a means to adhere to organisational policy rather than to improve practice (Anka et al, 2020; Gillingham, 2016). Practitioners also reported that digital technology did not align with the complexities of safeguarding practice (Broadhurst et al 2010; French and Stillman, 2014).

More recently, children safeguarding practice reviews have shown that digital technology presents challenges for safeguarding practice around practitioners' abilities to discern and assess the full extent of risks (CSPRP, 2022). To give one example, concerns have been raised about whether those who pose a risk are present during video interactions. Further, the literature identifies that while providing opportunities to connect with others, digital technology usage – including remote/hybrid working – has also resulted in less-supportive teams. Jeyasingham and Devlin (2024) note that remote working has had negative impacts on less-experienced staff (both newly qualified and those in training). This concurs with the findings of Thacker et al (2020), who note that remote working negatively impacts those who are less curious, as the opportunity to learn from more senior colleagues is limited when people work from home.

You need curiosity to discern what is going on when using digital technology in safeguarding work. A scoping review of the literature undertaken by Behan-Devlin (2024) on the use of digital technology in children's safeguarding social work practice found that although digital technology is now common practice, most of the research studies in this area have focused primarily on practitioners' perspectives rather than families' perspectives about such use. The recent literature tells us about artificial intelligence (AI) and its potential use to support practice. While this is good, the evidence base supporting use of AI in safeguarding practice is limited. Behan-Devlin (2024, p 2964) found that limited studies exist on the use of algorithmic decision-making tools that are trained in handling *'larger, more complex datasets, including information recorded by practitioners in EISs, in addition to "learning" to better calculate risk'*. The findings correspond with Ylönen's (2023, p 575) study, where it was noted that practitioners lacked training on using electronic information systems (EIS) which then led to more *'recording data instead of utilising it for professional purposes'*. Analysis of relevant SARs has identified a lack of recordings of case history and recommends improvement in case recordings. Practitioners report that most of the digital tools used to record assessments of risk are process driven and limit narrative description and analysis of family circumstances. This is corroborated by research. In Behan-Devlin's (2024) study, the findings across the papers reviewed recommended that practitioners should be involved in the design of electronic information systems to enable effective use of electronic information systems.

You learnt in Chapter 1 that being curious relates to a desire to learn. The increased use of digital technology and the issues highlighted create opportunities for individual practitioners and agencies to collaborate in research studies to find out more about how to harness and effectively use digital technology in safeguarding work. The British Association of Social Workers (BASW, 2018) draws attention to some of the benefits of digital technology, indicating that among other elements, dedicated interactive safeguarding apps in social care allow for self-reporting, immediate responses and access to information. This allows the opportunity for engagement in professional curiosity practice; it also provides the opportunity to examine practice in more depth. For example, this includes the ways people provide self-reports (the number of times, silence and non-reporting, what information is being accessed and who is accessing the information). Use of digital technology also provides an opportunity to apply legal literacy relating to information-sharing and data protection.

In safeguarding practice, while digital technology offers the opportunity to connect with others, it has also introduced new dangers and risks, such as the potential for scamming and financial abuse. You are required to use curiosity in your engagement with people using services so you can work with them to protect them from scamming. Good practice requires that you check and support people to use mobile devices rather than assume they will use them safely or that such devices are the only acceptable way to communicate. It is also important to check people's access to internet connections, as many rural locations still have poor internet access.

APPLYING CONCEPTS TO PRACTICE

Case study: learning from the SARs of 'Peter'

Multi-agency meetings regarding high-risk adults regularly discussed Peter. However, crucial information held by health practitioners on IV drug use and their concerns around acquired brain injury was not accessed by these agencies or shared with them. Limited data-sharing and the use of different systems appear to have created barriers and made it hard for frontline practitioners to know when there had been contact with other services and what form that took, affecting practice with Peter.

(Winter, 2021, p 18, 3.10)

TASK

- Make a list of how you would use digital technology to work with Peter.
- Work with a colleague from a different professional background who is also involved in safeguarding work. Write a draft risk plan of how your two agencies could work collaboratively with a service used in similar situation.
- Identify two potential challenges and explain how you and your colleagues might address these. Rewrite the draft risk plan and share with your team.
- Now read Peter's SAR (Winter, 2021) and identify one good practice that you would like to share with your team.
- Work with a colleague and prepare a peer learning presentation to your team on how to use MAST to help you and your team in a similar case.

Conclusion

This chapter has focused on the core skills, attributes and values underpinning professional curiosity and partnership work with those at the centre of safeguarding enquiries, their families and carers. The chapter also considered the skills required for partnership work with other professionals in the context of multi-agency and interdisciplinary work. It examined the concepts of empathy, critical thinking and analysis, and compassion and explored how these could be used to facilitate effective collaborative partnership work with people at risk or experiencing abuse, harm and neglect, and their families and carers. The chapter also considered new ways of working and the opportunities and challenges provided in using digital technology to connect with others, including practice implications. Case examples from SARs were used to illustrate some of the practice challenges and further learning. It is hoped that you can use the knowledge gained to inform your work with those at risk and those who are experiencing abuse, harm and neglect, their families and carers, and other professionals.

KEY POINTS FOR THIS CHAPTER

- 'Think person', 'think family', 'think collaboratively' by involving people, their families and carers as partners in safeguarding enquiries.
- Provide advocacy to enable those unable to participate in assessments and decision-making processes to participate.
- Involve people, their families and carers in assessing risks and co-create risk assessment and risk-enablement plans with them.
- Use empathy, critical thinking, analysis and compassion to understand the inner feelings of others and take action to alleviate their suffering.

- Showing empathy and compassion does not mean you take things at face value without appropriately examining information from different perspectives and exploring what is going on in more depth.
- Use digital technology to connect with others.
- Support those who are unable to use digital technology to do so (safely) by ensuring that the cost of digital technology is included in their personal budget.
- Strategic leaders and managers, including those supervising and supporting the learning of those in training (practice educators; practice supervisors and assessors), are urged to use empathy, critical thinking, analysis and compassion to work collaboratively with those on the front line and trainees.
- Strategic leaders should commission research on the use of AI for its potential benefit for promoting/enhancing collaborative and partnership work in safeguarding work and professional curiosity practice.

Further reading

Behan-Devlin, J (2024) Digital Technology in Children's Safeguarding Social Work Practice in the 21st Century: A Scoping Review. *The British Journal of Social Work*, 54(7): 2957–76. https://doi.org/10.1093/bjsw/bcae071.

Provides an overview about use of digital technology in safeguarding practice including impact.

Preston-Shoot, M, Braye, S, Doherty, C, Stacey, H, Hopkinson, P, Rees, K, Spreadbury, K and Taylor, G (2024) *Second National Analysis of Safeguarding Adult Reviews Final Report: Stage 2 Analysis of Learning*. [online] Available at: https://tinyurl.com/j6rv2t7f (accessed 13 November 2024).

Provides insights into lessons from SARs including good practice examples of how professional curiosity was used by practitioners.

Rawles, J (2023) Critical Thinking and Reflective Practice, in J Parker (ed), *Introducing Social Work*. London: Sage (pp 114–26).

Offers an accessible, easy-to-read perspectives on critical thinking.

Robinson, O C (2023) Probing in Qualitative Research Interviews: Theory and Practice. *Qualitative Research in Psychology*, 20(3): 382–397. https://doi.org/10.1080/14780887.2023.2238625.

Discusses different taxonomy of probe types; provides example questions on probing.

Santos Meneses, L (2020) Critical Thinking Perspectives Across Contexts and Curricula: Dominant, Neglected, and Complementing Dimensions. *Thinking Skills And Creativity*, 35: 100610. https://doi.org/10.1016/j.tsc.2019.100610.

Provides an overview of critical thinking. Discusses different dimensions, scope and presences of critical thinking through three movements.

7 Conclusion

> **CHAPTER OBJECTIVES**
>
> By the end of this chapter, you should be able to:
>
> - reflect on the key themes covered in the book;
> - consolidate and build on the learning gained from participation in the various activities and reflective tasks;
> - identify future learning priorities and develop an action plan to address these;
> - use the knowledge gained to inform your work with others;
> - use professional curiosity to safeguard those at risk or experiencing abuse, harm or neglect.

Introduction

This concluding chapter brings together the various topics discussed by drawing attention to the importance of using professional curiosity in safeguarding adult work. The chapter focuses on best practice and, in this light, has used selected examples of best practice from SARs to illustrate how you can use professional curiosity in the context of safeguarding adult practice. You are invited as a reader to consider ways in which professional curiosity lies at the centre of safeguarding adult work. You are also invited to reflect on your learning journey, to identify what you have learned including any future learning priorities and the key steps needed that will help you address these.

Best practice

As mentioned in the earlier chapters of this book, analysis of SARs identifies examples of best practice, although these are often outweighed by poor practice. Best practice refers to a positive way of doing something. Best practice is underpinned by evidence-based and value-based practice, is inclusive and places those at risk of or experiencing abuse, harm and neglect at the centre of practice. Citing Farkas and Anthony (2006), Osburn et al (2011, p 6) note that best practices *'are value-based practices that have recovery values underlying the practice'*. What follows looks at some examples of the best practice identified in SARs that relates to professional curiosity practice. Risk assessment is highlighted as one.

Risk assessments

Parker (2023, p 77) suggests that risk assessments relate to *'identifying, making clear and working to mitigate risks and dangers in the life choices and situations of those you work with'*. As mentioned in earlier chapters, risk assessments are central to safeguarding work. Development of competence in risk assessment is one of the key requirements of most professional qualifications, including social work (BASW, 2018; Social Work England (SWE) 2020), nursing and midwifery (Nursing and Midwifery Council, 2018) and policing (*Police and Criminal Evidence Act 1984*). Hilgartner (1992, p 41) uses the concept of risk to describe how *'things, situations or activities ... are seen as a source of danger'*. Other factors that impact the way risk is viewed or thought about can include culture, values and beliefs – hence the importance of using professional curiosity to unpick what the concept might mean to those at the centre of a safeguarding concern. This is in line with the principles underpinning the Making Safeguarding Personal policy and approaches discussed in Chapter 5. In safeguarding and professional curiosity practice, risk assessment involves identification, analysis and evaluation of risks that can increase harm, abuse and neglect. This includes potential as well as actual risks. Consistent with Making Safeguarding Personal principles, good risk assessment requires that you work with the person at the centre of safeguarding enquiry, their families and carers to understand their perceptions of risk and what they would like to see change. In the sample SARs selected, the best practices in risk assessments foregrounded good partnership work with the person and with other professionals, practitioners' use of person-centred, trauma-informed approaches, personalised responses and practitioners' persistence (Benbow, 2018; Oates, 2020; Spreadbury and Buckland, 2021; Rees, 2023; Preston-Shoot et al, 2024). In a SAR commissioned by Tower Hamlets Safeguarding Adults Board relating to adults with care and support needs and social isolation (Oates, 2020), best practices in risk assessments were achieved through good use of person-centred, personalised approaches and responses, including good partnership work with the adults themselves. What follows looks at the different stages involved in risk assessments consisting of risk identification, risk analysis and risk evaluation.

Risk-identification assessment

Risk-identification assessment should be informed by the categories of abuse outlined in the Care and Support Statutory Guidance (DHSC, 2024) discussed in Chapter 5. Here, the focus is to identify and describe the risks of harm, abuse and neglect, including potential and actual risks, care and support needs, unmet needs and potential impacts. It is also important to use the six principles underpinning safeguarding adults (also discussed in Chapter 5) to inform decision-making processes. A systematic review of the literature undertaken by NICE (2022), which sought to understand the approaches used by social workers to assess risks when working with adults with complex needs, recommended that assessments should facilitate open discussions about risks and understanding of different risks from different perspectives (including how risk is conceptualised by those at the centre of safeguarding concerns). NICE (2022) recommends that assessments should focus on risks relating to mortality and understanding of adverse events that require an immediate service response. In the context of professional curiosity practice, as discussed in Chapters 3, 4 and 6, it is very important to do everything in your capacity to build a relationship of trust with the individual. Preston-Shoot (2020) notes that key skills and approaches required for building relationships include taking a proactive rather than a reactive approach.

This book encourages you to use what Preston-Shoot (2020, p 6) describes as '*a combination of concerned and authoritative curiosity*', characterised by gentle persistence and '*work to build motivation with a focus on a person's fluctuating and conflicting hopes, fears and beliefs, and the barriers to change*'. Using such approaches provides the opportunity to explore the person's views, wishes, feelings and desired outcomes at a much deeper level. It also provides the opportunity to integrate and build on the person's strengths, capabilities and assets. As discussed in Chapter 6, some of the core skills and approaches required for carrying out risk assessments when using professional curiosity include intuition underpinned by cultural curiosity and culturally sensitive approaches, as using intuition alone runs the risk of judging the person in the light of our own assumptions and personal biases. You need to be self-aware of potential personal biases and use reflexivity and supervision to address these in line with the discussions in Chapters 2 and 3 (barriers and facilitators of professional curiosity). Tables 7.1, 7.2 and 7.3 provide risk-assessment and impact matrixes that you may use to assess potential and actual risks of harm, abuse and neglect. You are encouraged to use these in a co-productive way to construct the perceived and actual risk with the person at the centre of safeguarding concerns. For more reading on the use of risk assessment identification tools and templates, see Britten and Whitby (2018).

Table 7.1 Risk assessment and impact matrix

	Scores	Probability	Narratives description of risk	Action plan	By whom	Review of action plan	By whom
Likelihood	4	Almost certain					
	3	Probable					
	2	Possible					
	1	Hardly ever					

Table 7.2 Risk Assessment and Impact matrix

Impact		Low	Medium	High	Very high	Total scores	Action plan	By whom	By when	Review of action plan
Likelihood		(1)	(2)	(3)	(4)					
Where 5 is the highest	Almost certain (5)									
	Likely (4)									
	Possible (3)									
	Unlikely (2)									
	Rare (1)									
Impact scores x likelihood score = risk rating										

Table 7.3 Risk assessment and impact matrix

Narrative description of risk			By whom	Review of action to mitigate risk	Date reviewed
What could go wrong	What is working well	What can you put in place to mitigate risk			
Keep the voice of the personal central.					

Now consider the following case study.

APPLYING CONCEPTS TO PRACTICE

Case study

Jaspar is aged 40 and came to work in England from Tehran some years ago. He became May's partner two years ago. Jaspar has no other friends or social life. He moved in with May (aged 25) and her two children, Tim (four years) and Maggie (two years) a year ago. Tim has cystic fibrosis and Maggie appears to have developmental delays. The family lives in a one-bedroom local authority flat on the top floor of a tower block. The lifts frequently do not work and the flat is damp and cold due to the central heating not working. Jaspar has previously been diagnosed with bipolar disorder and his moods vary frequently. Jaspar refuses to take his prescribed medication due to the unpleasant side-effects. May has been looking after Jaspar during the past few weeks. The couple frequently shout and argue, and Jaspar has hit May several times. Over the last week, Jaspar has entered a manic phase of his illness and is hearing voices. He refuses to wash himself or his clothes. May visited her GP reporting feeling stressed and says this is due to looking after Jaspar and the children. You have received a call from a neighbour stating that Jaspar has locked himself in the bathroom threatening to kill himself.

TASK

- What key factors would you consider as potential and actual risks in this case scenario?
- Using the risk assessment and impact matrix, rate the likely impact of potential and actual risks identified.

- Consider how you would involve the family in this work.
- Who else would you involve and why?

Limitations of risk assessment impact matrix

It is worth pointing out that numerical grading is better suited in situations that are absolute. Examples of these include use in health settings or homes when assessing risks of falling, swallowing assessments or grade of pressure ulcers. It is important to know that, as with life, safeguarding work can be messy and it may not always be easy to capture all the issues and complexities of risk through a risk assessment impact matrix. Engagement in professional curiosity practice provides the opportunity for you to do so by asking curious questions about what might be missing. In such cases, you are encouraged to include a narrative description of the risk(s) identified and evaluate these in the wider context of overall risk to the individual.

Risk analysis

When employing professional curiosity, the risk analysis stage requires that you go beyond risk identification of potential and actual risks to a much deeper level by analysing the likely impact of the risks identified and considering an appropriate course of action. The risk analysis should include analysis of contextual factors (background, personal characteristics, intersectionality, capabilities, strengths and resources, personal assets) and their likely and actual impact on the person, their families and carers. This is supported by the NICE Review (2022) evidence relating to risk assessments. The Review recommended undertaking a thorough assessment of contextual factors that impact on the service user's life (NICE, 2022). Risk analysis also requires consideration of an appropriate course of action and resources needed to mitigate the risks identified including analysis of the likelihood of its potential and actual impact(s). To do so effectively, findings from the NICE Review (2022, p 16) noted that it is important to establish good communication between '*relevant service providers and people at risk and assessing risk in the context of people's broader lives*'. This leads us to the next stage – risk evaluation – but before doing so, consider this case scenario.

APPLYING CONCEPTS TO PRACTICE

Case study

Matthew is in his 60s, he is Turkish by racial ethnicity. Matthew has complex health care needs. He is currently homeless and sleeps at a local bus stop. You have received reports from members of the public that he defecates at the bus stop and there are empty cans of lager at the bus stop.

TASK

- What key factors would you consider as potential and actual risks in this case scenario?
- Using the Risk Assessment and Impact matrix (Table 7.2), rate the likely impact of potential and actual risks identified.
- Are there any risks relating to mortality and any adverse effects that may require an immediate service response? If so, who would you involve and why?
- How would you involve Matthew in this work?
- Now read the SAR on which this case scenario is based on and identify one good practice approach used by the professionals involved (SAR of MS, City of London and Hackney Safeguarding Adults Board, undertaken by Preston-Shoot, 2020).

In the SAR review of MS, the real situation which Matthew's case (above) is based on, the SAR report indicates that a number of agencies (eg housing, healthcare, police, fire service, adult social work and residential care nursing home practitioners) attempted to worked together to find solutions to address the risks (Preston-Shoot, 2020). The SAR report identified that MS was eventually placed in a residential care nursing home following a period of illness which resulted in a hospital admission (Preston-Shoot, 2020). Although the situation stabilised and there was improvement in his life while at the nursing home, things escalated (due to a number of safeguarding concerns around risks to self as well as risks to other residents and staff members) and MS ended up homeless and back on the street again (Preston-Shoot, 2020). This was a complex case which involved working with several competing rights and priorities (Preston-Shoot, 2020). In the SAR report, Preston-Shoot (2020) encourages practitioners to use person-centred, personalised approaches including trauma-informed approaches to work with people who may be caught up in similar situations. This corroborates with the NICE Review (2022), which also recommends using holistic, personalised approaches to risk assessments and analysis, facilitated by open conversations and shared decision making.

When faced with a similar situation, you might want to consider using integrative thinking to come up with possible creative solutions. Citing Martin (2009), Aven (2016, p2) suggests integrative thinking refers to the *'ability to face constructively the tension of opposing ideas and instead of choosing one at the expense of the other, generate a creative resolution of the tension in the form of a new idea that contains elements of the opposing ideas but is superior to each'*. What follows looks at risk evaluation and its importance in professional curiosity practice.

Risk evaluation

Risk evaluation involves appraisal, synthesis and analysis of the risk identified in a wider context of all the information obtained, including that gathered from all parties/agencies, the person at the centre of safeguarding concerns, their families and carers to inform the decisions to be taken. The risk-evaluation stage requires that you evaluate the risks in a wider context of law, policies and agency responsibilities in relation to the duties owed to protect a person's right to live free from abuse, neglect and harm (see Chapter 5 on the legal duties and human rights), including competing rights and imperatives. Risk evaluation should also include socio-economic and political factors that may impact the individual at the centre of safeguarding concerns as well as inter-agency resources and expertise. Evaluation of the risks identified should inform your decisions about an appropriate course of action and the resources required to mitigate and prevent the risks. Using professional curiosity underpinned by a critical reflexive approach will help you to examine your motivations, and those of your agency, particularly in relation to the decisions and actions taken to mitigate risks. It is also important to evaluate the risks in the wider contexts of inter-agency resources and expertise, and to draw from these to support the person at the centre of safeguarding concerns. Using professional curiosity would enable you to ask questions as well as find solutions to address issues/concerns relating to risk identified. Now consider the following case scenario.

APPLYING CONCEPTS TO PRACTICE
Case study

Zia, aged 50, lives with her son Jimmy, aged 23, and husband Robert, aged 63, in a three-bedroom house close to the city centre. The family are of White Russian descent. Robert has multiple sclerosis and now needs help with all personal care tasks; he is unable to manage on his own. He is supported by both Jimmy and Zia at home. Zia was diagnosed with bipolar depression shortly after Jimmy's birth and has previously had several compulsory admissions to psychiatric hospital but appears to be managing her situation with medication.

Jimmy is the main carer for both of his parents. He is studying to become a primary school teacher but has found it difficult to care for his parents. He has reported to the GP that he is under considerable strain as he has to wake up about four times during the night to attend to his father. With the family's consent, the GP referred Robert to Adult Social Services for assistance. Following the assessment, a care and support plan is put in place to support Robert. However, Zia has continued to find it difficult to accept that she now needs support from a stranger in order to help her care for her husband. Her mood has become very low and she is refusing to

> take her medication. Jimmy has noticed that his mother has not been attending to her personal care needs. He mentioned this to her this morning, but it resulted in an argument. He has received a phone call from the police that Zia has been found walking along the motorway calling for her mother (who died several years ago). The police report that Zia is confused; she doesn't appear to know where she is or have an awareness of her own safety.

TASK

- What are the safeguarding concerns raised in this case scenario?
- What contextual and intersectional factors impact the potential, actual and specific risks identified?
- What are the legal duties owed to Robert by the local authority?
- Under what legislation would an assessment of Jimmy and Zia's needs as carers be carried out?
- What curious questions would you ask?
- What resources are needed to address the issues identified?
- How would you use the resources to support the family?
- What constraints faced by your sector of practice are likely to impact on how you work with the family?
- What resources would you use to address the constraints faced (if any)?

As mentioned, risk evaluation also includes what services and support are available to promote risk management, as well as contingency plans that need to be put in place to address any fluctuating needs, uncertainties, surprises and other unforeseen issues. These should be informed and based on both evidence and a value-based approach. Table 7.4 provides an overview and a summary of the different stages of risk assessments discussed. Examples of best practice approaches identified in SARs are also provided after Table 7.4.

Table 7.4 Different stages of risk assessments

Risk identification **Evidence**	Use the categories of abuse outlined in the Care and Support Statutory Guidance accompanying the *Care Act 2014*. Include risks of suicide. Use Making Safeguarding Personal, trauma-informed and strengths-based approaches.

Risk analysis Knowledge base	Focus on analysis of contextual factors (personal characteristics, age, disabilities, gender, beliefs, sexuality, race). Fluctuations in risks. Resources (strengths-based, assets and capabilities). Use the six principles underpinning safeguarding adults. Think person, think carers, think family, think culture.
Risk evaluation	Evaluate risks in the wider contexts of: • socio-economic/political factors • legal/policy agency resources and practice approaches • inter-professional work, collaborations and partners (including expertise, specialist knowledge and inter-agency resources).
Action plan decisions	Decisions should be informed by evidence-based and value-based practice. Co-produced action plans with people with lived experiences and their advocates. Informed by compassion, empathy and risk-enablement plans. Supported by organisation resources, including in the wider community.

Best practice: trauma-informed approaches

Chapters 3 and 4 discussed what is meant by trauma and the importance of using trauma-informed approaches. Understanding the impact of trauma and the ability to use trauma and psychological-informed or trauma-aware approaches to engage with individuals at risk or who have experienced abuse, harm and neglect have been highlighted in SARs as best practice. Research on trauma-informed practice suggests that to work effectively with those who have experienced trauma, practitioners need to develop an understanding of the causes and components of trauma, their potential impacts and resultant trauma reactions (Senker et al, 2023). SARs demonstrate that the practitioners who use trauma-informed approaches are those who are able to sustain prolonged engagement with the people at the centre of safeguarding concerns (Rees, 2023; Spreadbury and Buckland, 2021). To reduce the risk of traumatisation and retraumatisation of those who have had or are experiencing traumatic stress-related difficulties, consideration should be given to the use of personalised and co-produced interventions that support the person's needs and outcomes. To work effectively with a person who has survived trauma, you will need to establish a safe space and give the person sufficient time. You also need to work towards reducing the likelihood and impact of trauma symptoms such as flashbacks and dissociation. The use of grounding skills to support the person to stay in the moment will help to increase their 'window of tolerance' – the zone of arousal in which a person is able to function most effectively (Seigal, 2020). When people are within this zone, they are typically able to readily receive, process and integrate information, and otherwise respond to the demands of everyday life without much difficulty, where they are not impacted by a fight, flight or freeze reaction (Seigal, 2020). For those who have experienced trauma in the past, SARs tell us that adopting an individualised flexible approach or using a person-centred approach can help to build trust and sustain engagement. This includes using individualised flexible approaches that support individuals who may find it difficult to engage with scheduled agency appointments to engage. In the SAR of the circumstances around the death of five women, Spreadbury and Buckland (2021) recommended considerations for using open-access or 'drop-in arrangements' to allow those unable to attend scheduled appointments to access support in their own time. What follows looks at examples of best practice relating to the use of personalised trauma-informed approaches.

Best practice in using personalised trauma-informed approaches

In the SAR of James, commissioned by Teeswide Safeguarding Adults Board, it was reported that James was born deaf and lived most of his life in foster care and residential care settings (Rees, 2023). James died at the age of 32. He was supported by a number of services. It was reported that James required support for alcohol and substance misuse. The SAR report also indicates that James was diagnosed with anxiety and depression and had a history of suicidal ideation/attempts; he was also a victim of sexual assault (Rees, 2023). James' family and carer (fiancée) described him as caring and as someone who put others first. James was placed in a shared housing facility when private accommodation arranged by a friend fell through. Rees (2023) reported that James didn't fit into the new household as the other housing tenants did not like James playing loud music late into the night (James had hearing difficulties and it was the only way he could listen to the music). Although James contributed to joint food shopping, the food bought was not food that James liked. Findings from the SAR identified several good practices. The report observes that *'there were several responses by agencies to questions regarding adapting care to a trauma-informed response'* (Rees 2023, p 7). There was evidence to suggest that James engaged well with practitioners when trauma-informed approaches were used. Rees (2023) noted that practitioners knew James needed two hearing aids but only used one due to an ear infection and they made reasonable adjustments by communicating in a way that enabled James to understand what was being said. The SAR report also noted that James found it difficult to attend appointments at the GP surgery due to his disabilities, but one practitioner changed the appointment settings to accommodate James and thus enabled him to attend appointments (Rees, 2023). This practitioner recognised that attending appointments at specific times and/or at agency settings conducive to the needs and outcomes of the person at the centre of safeguarding enquiry was more effective in engaging with James, so they acted on it and put this into practice. This aligns with the legal duties to make reasonable adjustments under section 20 of the *Equality Act 2010*, discussed in Chapter 5. The SAR report also indicates that James engaged particularly well in healthcare practices where he was not asked to retell his story. These included appointments at a diabetic clinic, with dietitians and at his GP surgery for blood tests. Rees (2023) noted the challenges this presents for professional disciplines – for example, in mental health, addiction and social care services where detailed information about personal histories is required to enable practitioners to gain a fuller picture of contextual factors likely to impact on and/or exacerbate risks to harm, abuse and neglect, such as the personal characteristics and contextual factors discussed in earlier chapters. In such situations, in line with the earlier discussion on the importance of multi-agency, inter-professional work, you may want to consider undertaking joint visits with other practitioners with whom the person at the centre of safeguarding concerns finds it easier to work and learning from key strategies used that make it easier to engage with the person. Joint visits are helpful ways to gather important information about what might be going on in the person's life. You can take notes while your colleague is talking to the person (or vice versa). Other approaches are using a key worker, a named person with whom the person gets on well, as the key coordinator or contact and to whom all referrals and contact with the person are made, and reporting back to the inter-agency, inter-professional team regarding the person, as mentioned earlier.

As mentioned previously, safeguarding work is complex and may require different expertise and resources to be pulled together to mitigate and address risks of harm, abuse and neglect. As discussed in previous chapters, it is not uncommon for different professionals to be involved in supporting the person at the centre of a safeguarding enquiry. Research identifies poor practice in inter-agency and interprofessional practice (around 95 per cent of the cases analysed in the second analysis of SARs in England) relating to poor coordination and communication (Preston-Shoot et al, 2024). Developing skills in coordinating assessments in interprofessional and inter-agency contexts is important to support individuals. Research identifies that safeguarding assessments can be intrusive and assessment processes that require those at the centre of safeguarding enquiries to retell their stories multiple times can lead to retraumatisation and should be undertaken with high levels of care and sensitivity. In addition to carrying out a joint visit with other professional colleagues, to mitigate the retelling of painful stories/histories consideration should be given to using different tools which can be shared (with the person's consent) with other professionals at different appointments. Personal information documents such as a 'healthcare passport', 'This is Me' or 'personal profile', such as those developed by the Alzheimer's Society (2021) to record important information, can be used to record information to allow the sharing of information between different settings in order to avoid retraumatising the person by asking them to retell their story.

The personal information document should draw from life story principles by including essential information about the person's life history, wishes and preferences, aspirations and desired outcomes, including how the person would like to be supported. It is important that all efforts are made to ensure the document is co-produced. Family members, carers and advocates should be involved in supporting those who are unable to tell their stories about what is important to them and consulted on how they would like to be supported to do so. In the SAR of James, Rees (2023) recommends that practitioners could use 'This is Me', a personal information document. 'This is Me' has been used successfully in dementia care and in work with people with learning disabilities to record important personal information about individuals' lives so the person does not have to constantly retell their story. Baillie and Thomas's (2020) research study affirmed the important use of personal information documents with those with communication challenges within dementia care. The authors found personal information documents were useful for capturing important information about the person living with dementia, which was then shared with other professionals at different settings (Baillie and Thomas, 2020). Personal information documents enable the voices of people with lived experience to be included in their care delivery, with their permission, without having to retell their stories repeatedly at different appointments and/or in different care settings.

Another useful tool (also from dementia care) that could be adapted for recording personalised information about those at the centre of safeguarding enquiries is 'Know Me', which is a digital toolkit. Using digital technology to connect with others was discussed in Chapter 6. The 'Know Me' digital toolkit provides an opportunity to record digitalised personalised co-produced risk-minimisation or risk-enablement care plans with individuals about whom there are safeguarding adult concerns. The toolkit is designed to capture information in four key domains: capability card, co-design guide, data exploration guide and person-centred canvas (Wang et al, 2021). Practitioners can use the toolkit to capture information about the person's capabilities (what they can do) and limitations (challenges – what they find it difficult to do) to inform intervention plans that focus on what can be done to address the challenges as well as build on the person's capabilities. Adopting a professional curiosity practice when co-creating the capabilities cards offers the opportunity to explore key factors that facilitate or hinder the person's capabilities. The use of such digital toolkits aligns with the earlier discussions about the importance of harnessing digital technology in safeguarding work (discussed in Chapter 6). Another useful tool that you could use to coordinate inter-agency risk assessment is the electronic health information exchange platform. This allows health and social care practitioners to share information effectively. Use of health information exchange has been commented on positively in analysis of several SARs as good practice in bringing different professionals together to coordinate assessment and risk-management plans that support those at risk of abuse, harm and neglect. As noted, though, it is also important to use professional curiosity to analyse and evaluate potential and actual risks posed by advancements in digital technology and usage in the context of safeguarding people from online abuse. Brookfield et al (2024) draw attention to the rise in technology-facilitated domestic abuse. These authors note that current risk-assessment tools used in safeguarding practice – Domestic Abuse, Stalking, Harassment and Honour Based Violence Assessment (DASH) and Multi Agency Risk Assessment Conference (MARAC) – do not fully allow the new dangers posed by digital technology in cases of domestic violence to be captured fully (Brookfield et al, 2024). This corroborates the work of Yardley (2020) and includes cases where perpetrators have used digital technology to track and or monitor victims/survivors' movements online, through social media and the use of smart home devices (Brookfield et al, 2024). As mentioned in earlier chapters, professional curiosity is about learning and having a learning mindset, including taking on new challenges.

> **APPLYING CONCEPTS TO PRACTICE**
>
> **Case study**
>
> Imagine that you are working in a multi-agency safeguarding adults' hub. Your team uses a number of risk assessments tools to assess and support service users. This includes an AI automated interactive desktop and mobile application system that enable service users to book appointment as well as seek support throughout the day and at weekends. The AI chatbots can answer common questions and provide guidance on a range of topics.

TASK

- What are your views about the use of AI in safeguarding adult practice?
- Make a list of potential advantages and draw backs of using AI in professional curiosity and safeguarding adult practice.
- Carry out an audit of the risk assessment tools used by your team, include any inter-agency/multi-professional assessment tools used to identify whether the tools allow practitioners to assess potential and actual risks posed by digital technology in assessments.
- Identify good practice and gaps in practice and report your findings to your team.

Rapport-building and persistence

SAR reports have highlighted the positive impact of rapport-building and being persistent. The discussion of the four types of curious people (Chapter 1) indicates that 'fascinators' possess an unwavering commitment to learn and are persistent in achieving their goal(s). Persisting in the face of challenges and setbacks and co-productively finding ways to work with an individual at the centre of a safeguarding enquiry to overcome the challenges is identified as good practice. SARs have identified that having the motivational endurance to persist, particularly when support is refused, and finding a way to enable support to be accepted, are central to sustaining engagement.

The concept of persistence is linked to the notion of perseverance – the act of being determined and the ability to keep going in the face of adversity or setbacks. The act of being persistent or persevering is described in the literature as a continuing goal orientation personality trait, characterised by the ability to continue to work towards a goal. It is argued that persistence and perseverance predispose a person to work towards a goal even in the face of adversity and or hardship. Writing from the perspective of student learning, Tinto (2017, p 2) views persistence as a *'quality that allows someone to continue in pursuit of a goal even when challenges arise'*. Adversities that are likely to be encountered in safeguarding work, as discussed in Chapter 2 on barriers to professional curiosity, can include the impact of listening to trauma narratives and/or exposure to traumatic environments, working with limited resources, organisational cultures and leadership.

The literature has identified that context affects practice. As discussed in Chapter 2, the structural systems and processes that frame ways of work, and the working environment, can also have an effect on our readiness and ability to be professionally curious. Self-regulation, self-direction and self-efficacy are identified as central to the ability to persist in the face of adversity. Some of the good practice examples drawn from SARs demonstrate that practitioners who showed unwavering commitment to working with the individuals by pursuing what worked for the individual rather than fitting the individual into existing systems and structures were more successful in sustaining engagement with the individual. In a SAR commissioned by Barnsley Safeguarding Adults Board relating to a 68 year-old man who died in a house fire, the author notes that *'the professional curiosity and resilience demonstrated by the officers attending resulted in them gaining access to the property having tried persistently for over an hour'* (Benbow, 2018, p 29, 6.6.1). The person referred to in the SAR report was called Jack. He lived on his own. It was reported that he had cooked on an open fire in his bedroom; a neighbour who witnessed smoke coming out of the house became concerned and checked on him. Reassurances were given by Jack that he had put the fire out and all was well. Unfortunately, Jack died in the house fire that night. A brief synopsis about Jack has been provided. You are now encouraged to read the full SAR report to gain an insight about who Jack was and how the different professionals worked together to support Jack. You are also encouraged to reflect on ways you might use professional curiosity to work with other people with similar challenges to Jack. From reading the full SAR, you would gather that Jack had complex health and social care needs but was reluctant to work with professionals and that he did not like professional intrusion into his life (Benbow, 2018).

It is important to note here that it was not just professionals who used curiosity in their engagement with Jack. In Jack's case, the neighbour also used curiosity and sought to find out what was going on in Jack's house when he saw the smoke and checked on Jack. Chapter 4 briefly touched on the notion of seeing safeguarding as 'everyone's business', as stipulated in policy. You learnt about the dangers of viewing 'professional curiosity' as something that only 'professionals do' and were encouraged to view professional curiosity similar to the policy agenda in safeguarding work as being 'everybody's business' in that chapter. It is important to note that curiosity is about showing interest; it is about having the permission to be nosy, to ask questions in a thoughtful, compassionate way.

You are encouraged to involve people, family, friends, carers and neighbours in professional curiosity and safeguarding work. Using professional curiosity would enable an effective risk assessment to be undertaken, allowing the opportunity to identify those who are well placed and able to assist the person at the centre of the safeguarding enquiry and those likely to exploit them. Such an approach allows the practitioner to build on people's strengths. In Jack's situation, the neighbours described him as loving animals; people in the community knew that they would find their missing pets at Jack's house when they went missing. While this was one of the key factors initiating professional involvement in Jack's life, you might want to consider how you could harness Jack's love of animals to involve and connect him with community projects in his neighbourhood. It is important to remember that Jack had legal rights. The legal and policy contexts of safeguarding work were considered in Chapter 5. The chapter included the legal obligations to save lives in line with the *Human Rights Act* (Article 2 – the right to life) and the right to protect people to live free from abuse, neglect and harm, as well as the rights to participation as enshrined in the *Care Act 2014*. Chapter 5 also included discussions of other legislative frameworks such as the *Mental Health Act* and *Mental Capacity Act*. In addition to the legal obligations to save lives, this book has considered the central importance of empathy and compassion in safeguarding work and the need to be persistent in using all the tools and resources available to effect and maintain change.

Other good practice recommendations found in SARs include suggestions to support outreach agencies that know the individual at the centre of safeguarding concern to be the key agency connect (maintain contact) with the individual and then report back to the whole multi-agency team (Preston-Shoot et al, 2024).

The role of managers and organisations

We considered the role of managers and organisations in Chapter 3. While most of the discussions in this book have centred on individual frontline practitioners and those training to work in safeguarding adults practice, SARs tell us that frontline practitioners and those in training cannot participate in professional curiosity practice without the support of their managers and organisations. The literature in this area indicates that effective professional curiosity practice is underpinned by effective strategic leadership, including successful commissions and the involvement and inclusion of the voices of people with lived experiences in decision-making (Preston-Shoot et al, 2024; Thacker et al, 2020). In the second national analysis of SARs in England, discussed previously, the authors reported that although there were positive observations relating to staff support, supervision and management oversights, most of the factors that had negative impacts on practice related to staffing levels and workloads (27 per cent), lack of management oversight (31 per cent) and gaps in commissioned service provision (24 per cent). In Chapter 6, it was stressed that if you experience any of these factors/issues, it is imperative to bring these concerns to your managers and strategic leaders' attention. For those in training, this may present a challenge. Managers are encouraged to create a safe, open work environment that enables those in training as well as practitioners to raise concerns as well as share good practice.

Conclusion

The book has focused on the concept of professional curiosity and the importance of using professional curiosity in safeguarding work, including the skills, attributes and behaviours required for professional curiosity practice. The earlier chapters introduced the concept of curiosity and professional curiosity in safeguarding, identifying challenges in definitions. As discussed, while different definitions of what is meant by professional curiosity exist from practitioners' perspectives, limited literature exists on what the concept means from people with lived experience. However, although this appears to be the case, like the perspectives offered from the practice literature – which mainly centres on skills, attributes and behaviour required for practice – PWLE also viewed professional curiosity as a skill required for practitioner involvement in safeguarding work. As also discussed, the concept of professional curiosity is conceptualised from the perspectives of PWLE as the practitioner's ability to use smart thinking and wondering questions to unpick what might be going on within complex family dynamics. Professional curiosity was also viewed from the perspectives of PWLE as a useful skill required to question as well as to challenge attitudes of professional dangerousness, as failing to ask appropriate questions could further place someone at risk of continuing harm, abuse and neglect. Professional curiosity was also viewed from the perspectives of people with lived experience as a tool to promote trust, allowing the opportunities to implement trauma-informed interventions that prevent and mitigate risk as well as to support resilience in families.

The book has highlighted the importance of professional curiosity in safeguarding adults practice, including the skills, knowledge and values required to use professional curiosity. As multiple SAR reviews have shown, a lack of professional curiosity is a key factor that led to the serious harm and death of those analysed within the SAR and who were owed the duty of protection from abuse, harm and neglect. Stevens et al (2022, p 11) identify curiosity as one of the '7 Cs' – attributes important to adult safeguarding alongside *'care, compassion, courage, communication, commitment [and] competence'*. Preston-Shoot (2017) describes professional curiosity as a critical skill for safeguarding adult practice. Stevens et al (2022) proposes that the practitioner needs curiosity to better understand, support and protect adults at risk of abuse and harm. As discussed in this book, safeguarding adults is complex; safeguarding means different things to different people. Safeguarding adults work cuts across different disciplines and diverse agencies are usually called on to find workable solutions to support the person and/or the families central to safeguarding concerns. Different professions may have differing approaches on how to protect the rights of people to live safely, free from abuse, harm and neglect. While these differences exist, it is important to note that safeguarding adults work encompasses key actions taken to protect and enable someone to live safely from abuse, harm and neglect. Safeguarding adult practice involves first seeing the person behind the safeguarding concerns as a human being and working from their perspectives about what it means to be safe to assist them. It requires practitioners to use professional curiosity to unpick what being safe means to the person, their families and carers, and what they want change to help them to feel safe. Examples drawn from analysis and learning from the human stories – both told and untold from SARs – have been used throughout this book to show the importance of using professional curiosity to safeguard adults. Learning from SARs has also been used to shed light on the consequences of failing to use professional curiosity when working with those at risk of, or experiencing, abuse, harm and neglect. This book has also drawn from the broad literature, research, law, policy, values and observations from practice and used these to make the case for why professional curiosity is so important in safeguarding work.

What is most important to us as authors is that you will use the knowledge and skills gained to work with others, including those at the centre of safeguarding enquiries, their families and carers, to save lives. Most of the learning drawn from SARs included in the previous chapters has highlighted practice that did not go as well as what did go well. As mentioned in earlier chapters, professional curiosity practice, and indeed SARs, foreground our learning in this area. The activities and reflective questions used in the book have sought to encourage you to participate in additional reading and tasks to enable you to gain further insights into what could be done in your safeguarding work.

The central argument throughout this book is that you have a professional mandate to ask curious questions to promote and protect the rights of people to live safely, free from abuse and neglect. The book has also argued that a focus on the legal mandate alone is not enough. Being professionally curious requires engaging with the person at the centre of safeguarding concerns on a human-to-human basis, using your skills and drawing from values that facilitate an enabling environment conducive to the needs and outcomes of the person at risk of harm, abuse and neglect. Professional curiosity practice also requires taking a compassionate approach, supported by inter-agency resources and expertise to enable the person, their families and carers to exercise their rights to live freely from abuse, neglect and harm. As authors, it is our hope that you have found this book helpful in allowing you to learn about professional curiosity and the practice skills needed to use curiosity when working with those at the centre of safeguarding enquiries, as well as in your work with other professionals. It is also our hope that you have taken (or can take) the necessary steps to seek any further training needed to address any gaps in knowledge, skills and attributes identified.

As with any other book, there are inevitable gaps in content. As authors, we took an interdisciplinary, interprofessional approach by writing for both those in training and practitioners with responsibilities for safeguarding adults. While this has provided the opportunity to examine some of the concepts of professional curiosity from a broader perspective, it has meant that the book has not been able to provide in-depth discussions on disciplinary specific practice issues and or concerns. It is our hope that the reflective activities, particularly those drawn from SARs, have provided specific disciplinary issues from which your profession needs to learn. It is also our hope that you are able to learn from the distinctive issues relating to interprofessional/inter-agency context raised in the SARs relating to professional curiosity practice. Further, although the book has primarily focused on England, it has international relevance: practitioners outside England can use the content to inform their practice, considering their own local and national policies and law. It is our hope that you will use the knowledge gained to effect change.

KEY POINTS FOR THIS CHAPTER

The chapter underscores the importance of:

- using professional curiosity in safeguarding adult work and the likely consequences of failing to do so;
- involving people at the centre of safeguarding enquiries in risk-identification assessments and decisions about what needs to be done to make them feel safe and in co-creating interventions that meet their desired outcomes;
- using different tools and frameworks to assess, analyse and evaluate potential and actual risks of harm, abuse and neglect. Examples include the use of risk assessment and impact matrix and personalised trauma-informed approaches;
- being persistent and not giving up in the face of adversities in your practice and learning;
- actively participating and reflecting on the knowledge gained, and seeking out further learning to inform your practice.

Further reading

Brookfield, K, Fyson, R and Goulden, M (2024) Technology-facilitated Domestic Abuse: An Under-recognised Safeguarding Issue?, *The British Journal of Social Work*, 54(1): 419–36. https://doi.org/10.1093/bjsw/bcad206.

Considers advancement in digital technology, including the impact of safeguarding adults risk-assessment tools.

Preston-Shoot, M (2020) *MS: A Safeguarding Adult Review*. London: City of London and Hackney Safeguarding Adults Board. [online] Available at https://tinyurl.com/4zav5c7v (accessed 13 November 2024).

Provides recommendations on good practice with those facing multiple-exclusion homelessness.

References

Adult with Incapacity (Scotland) Act 2000. [online] Available at: www.legislation.gov.uk/asp/2000/4/contents (accessed 13 November 2024).

Adult Support and Protection (Scotland) Act 2007. [online] Available at: www.legislation.gov.uk/asp/2007/10/contents (accessed 13 November 2024).

Afful, I (2018) The Impact of Values, Bias, Culture and Leadership on BME Under-representation in the Police Service. *International Journal of Emergency Services*, 7(1): 32–59. https://doi.org/10.1108/IJES-05-2017-0028.

Ahuja, L, Price, A, Bramwell, C, Briscoe, S, Shaw, L, Nunns, M, O'Rourke, G, Baron, S and Anderson, R (2022) Implementation of the Making Safeguarding Personal Approach to Strengths-based Adult Social Care: Systematic Review of Qualitative Research Evidence. *The British Journal of Social Work*, 52(8): 4640–63. https://doi.org/10.1093/bjsw/bcac076.

Allen, M and Tsakiris, T (2018) The Body as First Prior: Interoceptive Predictive Processing and the Primacy of Self-models. In M Tsakiris and, H De Preester (eds), *The Interoceptive Mind: From Homeostasis to Awareness*. Oxford: Oxford University Press.

A Local Authority v AW [2020] EWCOP 24.

Alzheimer's Society (2021) This is Me. [online] Available at: www.alzheimers.org.uk/get-support/publications-factsheets/this-is-me (accessed 13 November 2024).

Anka, A (2023) Social Work with Older People. In J Parker (ed), *Introducing Social Work*, 2nd ed. London: Sage.

Anka, A and Penhale, B (2024) Safeguarding Carers: Literature Review on What is Known About Carers Who are Abused by the People They Provide Care For. *The Journal of Adult Protection*, 26(3): 113–25. https://doi.org/10.1108/JAP-11-2023-0033.

Anka, A and Taylor, I (2016) Assessment as a Site of Power: A Bourdieusian Interrogation of Service User and Carer Involvement in the Assessments of Social Work Students. *Social Work Education*, 35(2): 17285. https://doi.org/10.1080/02615479.2015.1129397.

Anka, A, Thacker, H and Penhale, B (2020) Safeguarding Adults Practice and Remote Working in the COVID-19 Era: Challenges and Opportunities. *The Journal of Adult Protection*, 22(6): 415–27. https://doi.org/10.1108/JAP-08-2020-0040.

Anstiss, T, Passmore, J and Gilbert, P (2020) Compassion: The Essential Orientation. [online] Available at: https://tinyurl.com/njczsnxn (accessed 13 November 2024).

Asmussen, K, Fischer, F, Drayton, E and McBride, T (2020) Adverse Childhood Experiences: What We Know, What We Don't Know, and What Should Happen Next. [online] Available at: https://tinyurl.com/bdhk2h5x (accessed 13 November 2024).

Aven, T (2016) Risk Assessment and Risk Management: Review of Recent Advances on Their Foundation. *European Journal of Operational Research,* 253(1): 1–13. https://doi.org/10.1016/j.ejor.2015.12.023.

B v A Local Authority [2019] 3 WLR 685.

Baillie L, and Thomas, N (2020) Personal Information Documents for People with Dementia: Healthcare Staff's Perceptions and Experiences. *Dementia,* 19 (3): 574–89. https://doi.org/10.1177/1471301218778907.

Baginsky, M, Ixer, G and Manthorpe, J (2021) Practice Frameworks in Children's Services in England: An Attempt to Steer Social Work Back on Course? *Practice: Social Work in Action*, 33(1): 3–19. https://doi.org/10.1080/09503153.2019.1709634.

Bansal, A (2016) Turning Cross-cultural Medical Education on Its Head: Learning About Ourselves and Developing Respectful Curiosity. *Family Medicine and Community Health,* 4(2): 41–4. https://doi.org/10.15212/FMCH.2016.0109.

Barnett, D (2019) *The Straightforward Guide to Safeguarding Adults: From Getting the Basics Right to Applying the Care Act and Criminal Investigations*. London: Jessica Kingsley.

Barnsley Safeguarding Adult Board (2023) *Safeguarding Adult Review – Harry*. [online] Available at: https://tinyurl.com/bdfvx4em (accessed 13 November 2024).

Barrett, L F (2006) Solving the Emotion Paradox: Categorization and the Experience of Emotion. *Personality and Social Psychology Review,* 10(1): 20–46. https://doi.org/10.1207/s15327957pspr1001_2.

Barrett, L F (2017) The Theory of Constructed Emotion: An Active Inference Account of Interoception and Categorization. *Social Cognitive and Affective Neuroscience,* 12(1): 1–23. https://doi.org/10.1093/scan/nsw154.

Barrett, F L (2021) We Don't Understand How Emotions work. A Neuroscientist Explains Why We Often Get It Wrong. [online] Available at: https://tinyurl.com/2p9ppf9n (accessed 13 November 2024).

Bateman, F (2018) *Yi: A Safeguarding Adults Review, City and Hackney Safeguarding Adults Board*. [online] Available at: www.hackney.gov.uk/chsab-sars (accessed 13 November 2024).

Behan-Devlin, J (2024) Digital Technology in Children's Safeguarding Social Work Practice in the 21st Century: A Scoping Review. *The British Journal of Social Work,* 54(7): 2957–76. https://doi.org/10.1093/bjsw/bcae071.

Benbow, S M (2018) *Safeguarding Adult Review Jack*. Barnsley Safeguarding Adult Board. [online] Available at: https://tinyurl.com/5wxh2yuw (accessed 13 November 2024).

Berlyne, D E (1954) A Theory of Human Curiosity. *British Journal of Psychology,* 45(3): 180–91. https://doi.org/10.1111/j.2044-8295.1954.tb01243.x.

Bernard, H R (2013) *Social Research Methods: Qualitative and Quantitative Approaches*, 2nd ed. Thousand Oaks, CA: Sage.

Berry, A (2022) *Safeguarding Adult Review Overview Report Derek*, Oldham Safeguarding Adult Board. [online] Available at: https://tinyurl.com/57cuyapm (accessed 13 November 2024).

Boryczko, M (2022) Critical Thinking in Social Work Education: A Case Study of Knowledge in Students' Reflective Writing Using Semantic Gravity Profiling. *Social Work Education*, 41(3): 317–32. https://doi.org/10.1080/02615479.2020.1836143.

Botham, M (2024) *Local Child Safeguarding Practice Review (LCSPR) Child F*. Dudley Safeguarding People Partnership. [online] Available at: https://dudleysafeguarding.org.uk/wp-content/uploads/2024/03/LCSPR-Child-F-publication-date-27.03.24.pdf (accessed 13 November 2024).

Bottery, S and Mallorie, S (2024) *Social Care 360*. The Kings Fund. [online] Available at: www.kingsfund.org.uk/insight-and-analysis/long-reads/social-care-360 (accessed 13 November 2024).

Brabbs, C (2016) *Independent Overview Report of Mrs B*. Norfolk Safeguarding Adults Board. [online] Available at: https://tinyurl.com/4nt7n7pk (accessed 13 November 2024).

Braye, S, Orr, D and Preston-Shoot, M (2017) Autonomy and Protection in Self-neglect Work: The Ethical Complexity of Decision-making. *Ethics and Social Welfare*, 11(4): 320–35. https://doi.org/10.1080/17496535.2017.1290814.

Braye, S and Preston-Shoot, M (2020) *Safeguarding Adults Review of Mr A and Mrs A*. Leeds Safeguarding Adults Board. [online] Available at: https://tinyurl.com/av5exrmu (accessed 13 November 2024).

Britten, S and Whitby, K (2018) *Self-Neglect: A Practical Approach to Risk and Strengths Assessments*. St Albans: Critical Publishing.

Britten, S and Whitby, K (2021) *Self-Neglect Learning from Life*. St Albans: Critical Publishing.

British Association of Social Workers (BASW) (2014) *Code of Practice*. [online] Available at: https://tinyurl.com/muup9wvs (accessed 13 November 2024).

British Association of Social Workers (BASW), (2018) *Professional Capabilities Framework for Social Work: England Level descriptors for the four Pre-qualifying Levels and ASYE*. Birmingham: British Association of Social Workers.

Broadhurst, K, White, S, Fish, S, Munro, E, Fletcher, K and Lincoln, H (2010) *Ten Pitfalls and How to Avoid Them: What Research Tells Us*. National Society for the Prevention of Cruelty to Children. [online] Available at: https://tinyurl.com/xhz68eu3 (accessed 13 November 2024).

Brookfield, K Fyson, R Goulden, M (2024) Technology-facilitated Domestic Abuse: An Under-Recognised Safeguarding Issue?, *The British Journal of Social Work*, 54(1): 419–36. https://doi.org/10.1093/bjsw/bcad206.

Brookfield, S (1997) *Developing Critical Thinking*. Buckingham: Open University Press.

Burnard, P (1992) *Effective Communication Skills for Health Professionals*. London: Chapman and Hall.

Burton, V and Revell, L (2018) Professional Curiosity in Child Protection: Thinking the Unthinkable in a Neo-liberal World. *The British Journal of Social Work*, 48(6): 1508–23. https://doi.org/10.1093/bjsw/bcx123.

Calvard, T, Cherlin, E, Brewster, A and Curry, L (2023) Building Perspective-Taking as an Organizational Capability: A Change Intervention in a Health Care Setting. *Journal of Management Inquiry*, 32(1): 35–49. https://doi.org/10.1177/10564926211039014.

Care Act 2014. [online] Available at: www.legislation.gov.uk/ukpga/2014/23/contents (accessed 13 November 2024).

Care Quality Commission (2024) *The State of Health Care and Adult Social Care in England 2023/24.* [online] Available at: https://tinyurl.com/yzr4atxc (accessed 9 November 2024).

Chatfield, T (2018) *Critical Thinking: Your Guide to Effective Argument, Successful Analysis and Independent Study*. Thousand Oaks, CA: Sage.

Child Safeguarding Practice Review Panel (CSPRP) (2022) *Child Protection in England: National Review into the Murders of Arthur Labinjo Hughes and Star Hobson*. [online] Available at: https://tinyurl.com/yv9fehrh (accessed 13 November 2024).

Chu, L C (2024) Effect of Compassion Fatigue on Emotional Labor in Female Nurses: Moderating Effect of Self-compassion. *PLoS One,* 19(3): e0301101. https://doi.org/10.1371/journal.pone.0301101.

Clark, A (2023) *The Experience Machine.* Harmondsworth: Penguin.

Cocker, F and Joss, N (2016). Compassion Fatigue Among Healthcare, Emergency and Community Service Workers: A Systematic Review. *International Journal of Environmental Research and Public Health*, 13, 618. https://doi.org/10.3390/ijerph13060618.

Cooper, A, Lawson, J, Lewis, S and Williams, C (2015) Making Safeguarding Personal: Learning and Messages from the 2013/14 Programme. *Journal of Adult Protection*, 17(3): 153–65.

Córdova, A, Caballero-García, A, Drobnic, F, Roche, E and Noriega, D C (2023) Influence of Stress and Emotions in the Learning Process: The Example of COVID-19 on University Students: A Narrative Review. *Healthcare (Basel),* 11(12): 1787. https://doi.org/10.3390/healthcare11121787.

Cramphorn, K and Maynard, E (2023) The Professional in 'Professional Curiosity': Exploring the Experiences of School-based Pastoral Staff and Their Use of Curiosity with and About Parents. An Interpretative Phenomenological Analysis. *Pastoral Care in Education*, 41(1): 84–104. https://doi.org/10.1080/02643944.2021.1977989.

Criminal Law Act (Northern Ireland) 1967. [online] Available at: https://tinyurl.com/3t9xstpd (accessed 13 November 2024).

Croskerry, P (2013) From Mindless to Mindful Practice: Cognitive Bias and Clinical Decision Making. *The New England Journal of Medicine,* 368(26): 2445–8.

Cuff, B M P, Brown, S J, Taylor, L and Howat, D J (2016) Empathy: A Review of the Concept. *Emotion Review,* 8(2): 144–53. https://doi.org/0.1177/1754073914558466.

Data Protection Act 2018. [online] Available at: https://tinyurl.com/yc2hatbw (accessed 13 November 2024).

Davidson, G, Agnew, E, Brophy, L, Campbell, J, Donnelly, M, Farrell, A, Forbes, T, Frowde, R, Kelly, B D and McCartan, C (2024) Comparing Mental Health and Mental Capacity Law Data Across Borders: Challenges and Opportunities. *International Journal of Law and Psychiatry,* 92: 101949. https://doi.org/10.1016/j.ijlp.2023.101949.

Davis, J (2022) *Adultification Bias Within Child Protection and Safeguarding.* HM Inspectorate of Probation. [online] Available at: https://tinyurl.com/5k43av56 (accessed 13 November 2024).

Davis, J and Marsh, N (2020) Boys to Men: The cost of 'Adultification' in Safeguarding Responses to Black Boys. *Critical and Radical Social Work,* 8(2): 255–9.

Delgado, N, Delgado, J, Betancort, M, Bonache, H and Harris, L T (2023) What is the Link Between Different Components of Empathy and Burnout in Healthcare Professionals? A Systematic Review and Meta-Analysis. *Psychology Research Behavior Management,* 15(16): 447–63. https://doi.org/10.1016/j.ijlp.2023.10194910.2147/PRBM.S384247.

Department for Constitutional Affairs (2007) *Mental Capacity Act Code of Practice.* [online] Available at: www.gov.uk/government/publications/mental-capacity-act-code-of-practice (accessed 13 November 2024).

Department for Education (DfE) (2022) *CASPAR Briefing Summary of Serious Case Reviews 1998 to 2019: Continuities, Changes and Challenges.* [online] Available at: https://tinyurl.com/waerr5vt (accessed 13 November 2024).

Department of Health (2021) *Adult Protection Bill Consultation Analysis Report.* [online] Available at: https://tinyurl.com/22a9fdvt (accessed 13 November 2024).

Department of Health and Social Care (2019) *Strengths-based Approach: Practice Framework and Practice Handbook.* London: Department of Health and Social Care.

Department of Health and Social Care (DHSC) (2024) *Care & Support Statutory Guidance Issued under the Care Act 2014.* [online] Available at: https://tinyurl.com/yc566yad (accessed 13 November 2024).

Department of Health, Social Services and Public Safety (DHSSPS) and Department of Justice Adult (DoJ) (2015) *Safeguarding Prevention and Protection in Partnership.* [online] Available at: https://tinyurl.com/2exxv6kv (accessed 13 November 2024).

Depow, G, Francis, Z and Inzlicht, M (2021) The Experience of Empathy in Everyday Life. *Psychological Science,* 32(1). https://doi.org/10.1177/0956797621995202.

Dickens, J, Cook, L, Cossar, J, Okpokiri, C, Taylor, J and Garstang, J (2023) Re-envisaging Professional Curiosity and Challenge: Messages for Child Protection Practice from Reviews of Serious Cases in England. *Children and Youth Services Review,* 152: 107081. https://doi.org/10.1016/j.childyouth.2023.107081.

Dickens, J, Taylor, J, Cook, L, Cossar, J, Garstang, J, Harris, N, Molloy, E, Rennolds, N, Rimmer, J, Sorensen, P and Wate, R (2022) *Learning for the Future: Final Analysis of Serious Case Reviews 2017–19.* London: Department of Education. [online] Available at: https://scr.researchinpractice.org.uk (accessed 13 November 2024).

DL Va Local Authority and Others [2012] EWCA Civ 253. [online] Available at: www.casemine.com/judgement/uk/5a8ff6fe60d03e7f57ea5673 (accessed 13 November 2024).

Doherty, J (2024) *Local Child Safeguarding Practice Review Report Baby Y.* Bexley Safeguarding Partnership for Children and Young People (Bexley S.H.I.E.L.D.). [online] Available at: https://tinyurl.com/ah86ut7p (accessed 13 November 2024).

Domestic Abuse Act 2021. [online] Available at: www.legislation.gov.uk/ukpga/2021/17/contents (accessed 13 November 2024).

Domestic Abuse and Civil Proceedings Act (Northern Ireland) 2021. [online] Available at: https://tinyurl.com/mryjajra (accessed 13 November 2024).

Douglass, A (2016) *Mental Capacity: Updating New Zealand's Law and Practice.* Dunedin: New Zealand Law Foundation. [online] Available at: www.aspenltd. co.nz/mc/assets/Full_Report.pdf (accessed 13 November 2024).

Dyche, L and Epstein, R M (2011) Curiosity and Medical Education. *Medical Education,* 45(7): 663–68. https://doi.org/10.1111/j.1365-2923.2011.03944.x.

Efilti, P and Gelmez, K (2023) Mapping Three Dimensions of Empathy in Design Education: Educational Interventions, Aspects and Contexts. *Art, Design & Communication in Higher Education,* 22(1): 121–48. https://doi.org/10.1386/adch_00068_1.

Egan, G. (2018) *The Skilled Helper: A Problem-managements and Opportunity Development Approach.* Pacific Grove, CA: Brooks/Cole.

Equality Act 2010. [online] Available at: www.legislation.gov.uk/ukpga/2010/15/contents (accessed 13 November 2024).

Farkas, M and Anthony, W (2006) System Transformation Through Best Practices. *Psychiatric Rehabilitation Journal,* 30(2): 87–8. https://doi.org/10.2975/30.2006.87.88.

Featherston, R J, Shlonsky, A, Lewis, C, Luong, M L, Downie, L E, Vogel, A P, Granger, C, Hamilton, B and Galvin, K (2019) Interventions to Mitigate Bias in Social Work Decision-Making: A Systematic Review. *Research on Social Work Practice,* 29(7): 741–52. https://doi.org/10.1177/1049731518819160.

Feldon, P (2024) *The Social Worker's Guide to the Care Act 2014,* 2nd ed. St Albans: Critical Publishing.

Ferguson, H (2017) How Children Become Invisible in Child Protection Work: Findings from Research into Day-to-Day Social Work Practice. *The British Journal of Social Work,* 47(4): 1007–23. https://doi.org/10.1093/bjsw/bcw065.

Filipponi, C, Pizzoli, S F M, Masiero, M, Cutica, I and Pravettoni, G (2024) The Partial Mediator Role of Satisficing Decision-Making Style Between Trait Emotional Intelligence and Compassion Fatigue in Healthcare Professionals. *Psychological Reports,* 127(2): 868–86. https://doi.org/1010.1177/00332941221129127.

Fraga Dominguez, S, Storey, J E and Glorney, E (2022) Characterizing Elder Abuse in the UK: A Description of Cases Reported to a National Helpline. *Journal of Applied Gerontology,* 41(11): 2392–403. https://doi.org/10.1177/07334648221109513.

Frame, H (2017) *Safeguarding Adult Review: Adult C.* Nottinghamshire Safeguarding Adults Board. [online] Available at: https://tinyurl.com/2p846wzb (accessed 13 November 2024).

Freire, P (1998) *Pedagogy of Freedom: Ethics, Democracy, and Civic Courage.* Lanham, MD: Rowman and Littlefield.

French, R and Stillman, L (2014) The Informationalisation of the Australian community sector. *Social Policy and Society*, 13(4): 623–34. https://doi.org/10.1017/S1474746414000098.

Fynn, J F, Milton, K, Hardeman, W and Jones, A P (2022) A Model for Effective Partnership Working to Support Programme Evaluation. *Evaluation*, 28(3): 284–307. https://doi.org/10.1177/13563890221096178.

Garnett, A, Hui, L, Oleynikov, C and Boamah, S (2023) Compassion Fatigue in Healthcare Providers: A Scoping Review. *BMC Health Service Research*, 23(1): 1336. https://doi.org/10.1186/s12913-023-10356-3.

Garratt, K and Laing, J (2022) *Reforming the Mental Health Act.* House of Commons Library Research Briefing CBP-9132. [online] Available at: https://tinyurl.com/ekbxnxa8 (accessed 13 November 2024).

Gibson, J (2019) Mindfulness, interoception and the body: A contemporary perspective. *Neuropsychology,* 13(10): 2012. https://doi.org/10.3389/fpsyg.2019.02012.

Gilbert, P (2013) *The Compassionate Mind.* London: Constable Robinson.

Gillingham, P (2016) Technology Configuring the User: Implications for the Redesign of Electronic Information Systems in Social Work. *British Journal of Social Work*, 46(2): 323–38. www.jstor.org/stable/43905458.

Gorden, R L (1987) *Interviewing: Strategy, Techniques and Tactics,* 3rd ed. Homewood, IL: Dorsey Press.

Guthrie, L (2020) *Using a Systemic Lens in Supervision.* Totnes: Practice Supervisor Development Programme.

Hafford-Letchfield, T and Carr, S (2017) Promoting Safeguarding: Self-Determination, Involvement and Engagement in Adult Safeguarding. In A Cooper and E White (eds), *Safeguarding Adults Under the Care Act 2014: Understanding Good Practice.* London: Jessica Kingsley.

Hafford-Letchfield, T, Carr, S, Faulkner, A, Gould, D, Khisa, C, Cohen, R and Megele, C (2021) Practitioner Perspectives on Service Users' Experiences of Targeted Violence and Hostility in Mental Health and Adult Safeguarding. *Disability & Society*, 36(7): 1099–124. https://doi.org/10.1080/09687599.2020.1779033.

Hargie, O (2016) *Skilled Interpersonal Communication: Research, Theory and Practice.* London: Routledge.

Harvard Health Publishing (2020) *Understanding the Stress Response.* [online] Available at: https://tinyurl.com/2t7cv3zc (accessed 13 November 2024).

Health and Care Act 2022. [online] Available at: https://tinyurl.com/y2esu5ss (accessed 31 May 2024).

Hilgartner, S (1992) The Social Construction of Risk Objects: Or, How to Pry Open Networks of Risk. In J F Short and L Clarke (eds), *Organizations, Uncertainties, and Risk* (pp 39–53). Boulder, CO: Westview Press.

HM Government (2022) *Consultation on Proposed Changes to the Mental Capacity Act 2005 Code of Practice and Implementation of the Liberty Protection Safeguards Including the Liberty Protection Safeguards Secondary Legislation*. [online] Available at: https://tinyurl.com/2vw69k5n (accessed 13 November 2024).

HM Inspectorate of Probation (2022) *Practitioner: Professional Curiosity Insights Guide*. Manchester: HM Inspectorate of Probation. [online] Available at: www.justiceinspectorates.gov.uk/hmiprobation (accessed 13 November 2024).

Hopkinson, P (2023) *Safeguarding Adult Review of Brian: Swindon Safeguarding Partnership*. [online] Available at: https://tinyurl.com/mt9yvb78 (accessed 13 November 2024).

Human Rights Act 1998. [online] Available at: www.legislation.gov.uk/ukpga/1998/42/contents (accessed 13 November 2024).

Hutson, M (2023) *The Experience Machine Review: What the Brain Sees*. [online] Available at: https://tinyurl.com/mwfrvska (accessed 13 November 2024).

Isham, L, Bradbury-Jones, C and Hewison, A (2020) Female Family Carers' Experiences of Violent, Abusive or Harmful Behaviour by the Older Person for Whom They Care: A Case of Epistemic Injustice? *Sociology of Health & Illness*, 42(1): 80–94. https://doi.org/10.1111/1467-9566.12986.

Jackson-Best, F and Edwards, N (2018) Stigma and Intersectionality: A Systematic Review of Systematic Reviews Across HIV/AIDS, Mental Illness, and Physical Disability. *BMC Public Health*, 18: 919. https://doi.org/10.1186/s12889-018-5861-3.

Jeyasingham, D and Devlin, J (2024) Hybrid and Digitally Mediated Practice in Child and Family Social Work: Impacts on More and Less Experienced Practitioners' Communication, Relationships, Sense-Making and Experiences of Work. *The British Journal of Social Work*, 54(5): 2163–80. https://doi.org/10.1093/bjsw/bcae025.

Jones, D (2022) 10 minutes: Making 'Unwise' Decisions. *InnovAiT*, 15(8): 490. https://doi.org/10.1177/17557380211070028.

Kahneman, D (2011) *Thinking Fast and Slow*. Harmondsworth: Penguin.

Kashdan, T B, Stiksma, M C, Disabato, D J, McKnight, P E, Bekier, J, Kaji, J and Lazarus, R (2018) The Five-dimensional Curiosity Scale: Capturing the Bandwidth of Curiosity and Identifying Four Unique Subgroups of Curious People. *Journal of Research in Personality*, 73: 130–49.

Kedge, S and Appleby, B (2009) Promoting a Culture of Curiosity Within Nursing Practice. *British Journal of Nursing*, 18(10): 635–7. https://doi.org/10.12968/bjon.2009.18.10.42485.

Kemshall, H (2002) Effective Practice in Probation: An Example of 'Advanced Liberal' Responsibilisation? *The Howard Journal of Criminal Justice*, 41(1): 41–58.

Kidd, C and Hayden, B J (2015) The Psychology and Neuroscience of Curiosity. *Neuron*, 88(3): 449–60. https://doi.org/10.1016/j.neuron.2015.09.010.

King, S H Jr (2011) The Structure of Empathy in Social Work Practice. *Journal of Human Behavior in the Social Environment*, 21(6): 679–95. doi.org/10.1080/10911.

Kinman, G and Grant, L (2020) Emotional demands, compassion and mental health in social workers. *Occupational Medicine,* 70(2): 89–94. https://doi.org/10.1093/occmed/kqz144.

Korteling, J E and Toet, A (2020) Cognitive Biases. In S Della Sala (ed), *Reference Module in Neuroscience and Biobehavioral Psychology*. Amsterdam: Elsevier.

Ku, G, Wang, C S and Galinsky, A D (2015) The Promise and Perversity of Perspective-taking in Organizations. *Research in Organizational Behavior*, 35: 79–102. https://doi.org/10.1016/j.riob.2015.07.003.

Labour Party (UK) (2024) *Labour Party Manifesto 2024: Our Plan to Change Britain*, 13 June. [online] Available at: https://labour.org.uk/updates/stories/labour-manifesto-2024-sign-up (accessed 13 November 2024).

Lacy, R, Page, S and Wild, L (2021) *Safeguarding Adults Review in Rapid Time 'Issy'*. Richmond and Wandsworth Safeguarding Adults Board. [online] Available at: https://tinyurl.com/mu72dtbv (accessed 13 November 2024).

Laming, W H (2003) *The Victoria Climbie Inquiry: Report of an Inquiry*. London: The Stationery Office.

Lawless, M T, Marshall, A, Mittinty, M M and Harvey, G (2020) What Does Integrated Care Mean from an Older Person's Perspective? A Scoping Review. *British Medical Journal Open,* 10: e035157. https://doi.org/10.1136/bmjopen-2019-035157.

Leigh, J, Beddoe, L and Keddell, E (2020) Disguised Compliance or Undisguised Nonsense? A Critical Discourse Analysis of Compliance and Resistance in Social Work Practice. *Families, Relationships and Societies*, 9(2): 269–85. https://doi.org/10.1332/204674319X15536730156921.

Litman, J A (2008) Interest and deprivation factors of epistemic curiosity. *Personality and Individual Difference*, 44(7): 1585–95. https://doi.org/10.1016/j.paid.2008.01.014.

Litman, J A and Jimerson, T L (2004) The Measurement of Curiosity as a Feeling of Deprivation. *Journal of Personality Assessment*, 82(2): 147–57. https://doi.org/10.1207/s15327752jpa8202_3.

Litman, J A and Spielberger, C D (2003) Measuring Epistemic Curiosity and Its Diversive and Specific Components. *Journal of Personality Assessment,* 80(1): 75–86. https://doi.org/10.1207/S15327752JPA8001_16.

Lluch, C, Galiana, L, Doménech, P and Sansó, N (2022) The Impact of the COVID-19 Pandemic on Burnout, Compassion Fatigue, and Compassion Satisfaction in Healthcare Personnel: A Systematic Review of the Literature Published during the First Year of the Pandemic. *Healthcare*, 10(2): 364. https://doi.org/10.3390/healthcare10020364.

Local Government Association (LGA) and Association of Directors of Social Services (ADASS) (2019) *'Myths and Realities' About Making Safeguarding Personal*. London: LGA & ADASS.

Loewenstein, G (1994) The Psychology of Curiosity: A Review and Reinterpretation. *Psychology Bulletin,* 116(1): 75–98.

MacDonald, C (2024) *Sophia's Safeguarding Practice Review.* Northumberland Children and Adults Safeguarding Partnership. [online] Available at: https://tinyurl.com/mwdwxrx7 (accessed 13 November 2024).

Mallorie, S (2024) *Illustrating the Relationship Between Poverty and NHS Services.* The King's Fund. [online] Available at: https://tinyurl.com/5xaa4m7c (accessed 9 November 2024).

Malmedal, W (2020) If You Do Not Believe That It Happens You Won't See It Either! Sexual Abuse in Later Life. In A Phelan (ed), *Advances in Elder Abuse Research: International Perspectives on Aging* (pp 73–83). Cham: Springer.

Martin, K, Bickle, K and Lok, J (2022) Investigating the Impact of Cognitive Bias in Nursing Documentation on Decision-making and Judgement. *International Journal of Mental Health Nursing*, 31(4): 897–907. https://doi.org/10.1111/inm.12997.

Martin, R (2009) *The Opposable Mind*. Boston: Harvard Business Press.

Maynard, E and Cramphorn, K (2021) The Professional in Professional Curiosity: Exploring the Experiences of School-based Pastoral Staff and Their Use of Curiosity with and About Parents: An Interpretative Phenomenological Analysis. *Pastoral Care in Education,* 41(1)*:* 84–104. https://doi.org/10.1080/02643944.2021.1977989.

Mears, G. (2020) *Domestic Homicide Review into the Death of Daisy.* NCCSP. Available at: www.hundredfamilies.org/wp/wp-content/uploads/2022/04/MICHAEL-VIRGO-DHR-Full-July-2019.pdf (accessed 13 November 2024).

Mental Capacity Act 2005. [online] Available at: www.legislation.gov.uk/ukpga/2005/9/contents (accessed 13 November 2024).

Mental Capacity (Amendment) Act 2019. [online] Available at: www.legislation.gov.uk/ukpga/2019/18 (accessed 13 November 2024).

Mental Capacity Act (Northern Ireland) 2016. [online] Available at: www.legislation.gov.uk/nia/2016/18/contents/enacted (accessed 13 November 2024).

Mental Health Act 1983. [online] Available at: www.legislation.gov.uk/ukpga/1983/20/contents (accessed 13 November 2024).

Mental Health Act 2007. [online] Available at: www.legislation.gov.uk/ukpga/2007/12/contents (accessed 13 November 2024).

The Mental Health (Northern Ireland) Order 1986. [online] Available at: www.legislation.gov.uk/nisi/1986/595 (accessed 13 November 2024).

Miller, R, Glasby, J and Dickinson, H (2021) Integrated Health and Social Care In England: Ten Years On. *International Journal of Integrated Care,* 21(4): 1–9. https://doi.org/10.5334/ijic.5666.

Mlambo, M, Silén, C and McGrath, C (2021) Lifelong Learning and Nurses Continuing Professional Development; A Metasynthesis of the Literature. *BMC Nursing*, 20: 62. https://doi.org/10.1186/s12912-021-00579-2.

Moyle, S (2014) *Sine Wave Speech*. You Tube. [online] Available at: https://tinyurl.com/3fm6xtad (accessed 13 November 2024).

Muirden, C E and Appleton, J V (2022) Health and Social Care Practitioners' Experiences of Exercising Professional Curiosity in Child Protection Practice: An Integrative Review.

Health & Social Care in the Community, 30: e3885–e3903. https://doi.org/10.1111/hsc.14088.

Munro, E (2010) *The Munro Review of Child Protection Part One: A Systems Analysis.* [online] Available at: https://tinyurl.com/yeaxuw9y (accessed 13 November 2024).

National Wales Safeguarding Procedures (2021) *Wales Safeguarding Procedures.* [online] Available at: www.northwalessafeguardingboard.wales/wp-content/uploads/2020/06/Whats-Changed-Adults-Eng.pdf (accessed 13 November 2024).

National Institute for Health and Care Excellence (NICE) (2022) *Guideline NG216: Social Work with Adults Experiencing Complex Needs.* [online] Available at: www.nice.org.uk/guidance/NG216 (accessed 13 November 2024).

Newsam, S (2023) *Safeguarding Adults Review 'Riley'.* Tameside Safeguarding Adults Board. [online] Available at: https://tinyurl.com/2ukfmdvc (accessed 13 November 2024).

NHS Digital (2024a) Appointments in General Practice, April 2024. [online] Available at: GP_Appointment_Publication_Summary_April_2024.xlsx (live.com) (accessed 13 November 2024).

NHS Digital (2024b) *Safeguarding Adults Collection 2023–24.* [online] Available at: https://tinyurl.com/5n8nr7sa (accessed 13 November 2024).

NHS England (2023a) *2023/24 Priorities and Operational Planning Guidance.* [online] Available at: https://tinyurl.com/ut3u4dcv (accessed 20 June 2024).

NHS England (2023b) *Working in Partnership with People and Communities: Statutory Guidance.* [online] Available at: www.england.nhs.uk/publication/working-in-partnership-with-people-and-communities-statutory-guidance (accessed 13 November 2024).

Nicholls, P (2022) *Safeguarding Adults Review: Adults L, M & N.* Norfolk Safeguarding Adults Board. [Online] Available at: https://tinyurl.com/63fv3u8y (accessed 13 November 2024).

Nicolas, J (2016) Identifying Cases of Disguised Compliance. *Journal of Family Health*, 26(6): 27–32.

Norfolk Safeguarding Adults Board (2021) *Safeguarding Adults Review: Joanna, Jon & Ben.* [online] Available at: https://tinyurl.com/5hfdwd7w (accessed 13 November 2024).

Norfolk Safeguarding Adults Board (2022) *Professional Curiosity Guidance.* [online] Available at: www.norfolksafeguardingadultsboard.info/protecting-adults/working-with-adults-at-risk/professional-curiosity (accessed 13 November 2024).

Norfolk Safeguarding Adult Boards (2023) Seven-minute Briefing on Trauma-informed Approaches. [online] Available at: https://tinyurl.com/3x4kzvbe (accessed 13 November 2024).

Northamptonshire Safeguarding Adult Board (2023) *Safeguarding Adults Review (SAR) 024 – Adult A.* [online] Available at: https://staging-8939-westnorthantscouncil2.wpcomstaging.com/wp-content/uploads/2024/03/NSAB_S1.pdf (accessed 13 November 2024).

Nursing and Midwifery Council (2018) *The Code Professional Standards of Practice and Behaviour for Nurses, Midwives and Nursing Associates.* [online] Available at: https://tinyurl.com/3prv45jx (accessed 13 November 2024).

Oates, B (2020) *A Thematic Safeguarding Adult Review in Relation to Adults with Care and Support Needs and Social Isolation.* Tower Hamlets Safeguarding Adults Board. [online] Available at: https://tinyurl.com/4vaw6uct (accessed 13 November 2024).

Office for Health Improvement and Disparities (2022) *Guidance Working Definition of Trauma-informed Practice.* [online] Available at: https://tinyurl.com/mt6d45w3 (accessed 13 November 2024).

Oldham MBC v GW and PW [2007] EWHC 136 (Fam).

Okpokiri, C, Neil, E and Dhabha, A (2024) An Evaluation of Requisite Parenting – an Optimal Black Parenting Style. [online] Available at: https://tinyurl.com/yya638zj (accessed 13 November 2024).

Organisation for Security and Co-operation in Europe (OSCE) and Office for Democratic Institutions and Human Rights (ODIHR) (2023) Guidance on Trauma-informed National Referral Mechanisms and Responses to Human Trafficking. [online] Available at: www.osce.org/files/f/documents/1/9/549793.pdf (accessed 13 November 2024).

Osburn, O, Caruso, G and Wolfensberger, W (2011) The Concept of Best Practice: A Brief Overview of Its Meanings, Scope, Uses, and Shortcomings. *International Journal of Disability Development and Education,* 58(3): 213–22. https://doi.org/10.1080/1034912X.2011.598387.

Padesky, C and Mooney, K (1990) Clinical Tip Presenting the Cognitive Model to Clients. *International Cognitive Therapy Newsletter,* 6: 13–14.

Parker, J (2023) The Work Process: Assessment, Planning, Intervention and Review. In J Parker (ed), *Introducing Social Work.* London: Sage.

PC v City of York Council [2014] 2 WLR 1.

Percy-Smith, J (2006) What Works in Strategic Partnerships for Children: A Research Review. *Children and Society,* 20(4): 313–23. https://doi.org/10.1111/j.1099-0860.2006.00048.x.

PH v A Local Authority, Z Ltd and R [2011] EWHC 1704 (Fam).

Phillips, J, Ainslie, S, Fowler, A and Westaby, C (2022) What Does Professional Curiosity Mean to You? An Exploration of Professional Curiosity in Probation. *British Journal of Social Work,* 52: 554–72. https://doi.org/10.1093/bjsw/bcab019.

Phillips, J, Ainslie, S, Fowler, A and Westaby, C (2024). Lifting the Lid on Pandora's Box: Putting Professional Curiosity into Practice. *Criminology & Criminal Justice*, 24(2): 321–38. https://doi.org/10.1177/17488958221116323.

Police and Criminal Evidence Act 1984. [online] Available at: www.legislation.gov.uk/ukpga/1984/60/contents (accessed 13 November 2024).

Policy in Practice (2023) *Multi-Agency Safeguarding Tracker (MAST).* [online] Available at: https://policyinpractice.co.uk/mast (accessed 13 November 2024).

Poorkavoos, M (2016) *Compassionate Leadership: What is It and Why Do Organisations Need More of It?* Roffey Park Institute. [online] Available at: https://tinyurl.com/48525msm (accessed 13 November 2024).

Precey, M (2024) Suicidal Woman Repeatedly Called Funeral Firms. *BBC News*, 11 July. [online] Available at: www.bbc.co.uk/news/articles/ck55xw10xgyo (accessed 13 November 2024).

Preston-Shoot, M (2017) *What Difference Does Legislation Make? Adult Safeguarding Through the Lens of Serious Case Reviews and Safeguarding Adult Reviews*. Southwest Region Safeguarding Adults Boards. [online] Available at: https://tinyurl.com/2nxxwtve (accessed 2 July 2024).

Preston-Shoot, M (2020) *MS: A Safeguarding Adult Review*. City of London and Hackney Safeguarding Adults Board. [online] Available at: www.healthwatchhackney.co.uk/wp-content/uploads/2021/01/MS-SAR-Report-v3.2.docx.pdf (accessed 13 November 2024).

Preston-Shoot, M (2023) Human Stories About Self-neglect: Told, Untold, Untellable and Unheard Narratives in Safeguarding Adult Reviews, *The Journal of Adult Protection*, 25(6): 321–38. https://doi.org/10.1108/JAP-04-2023-0014.

Preston-Shoot, M, Braye, S, Doherty, C, Stacey, H, Hopkinson, P, Rees, K, Spreadbury, K and Taylor, G (2024) *Second National Analysis of Safeguarding Adult Reviews: Final Report*. [online] Available at: https://tinyurl.com/y2xnhm4p (accessed 13 November 2024).

Preston-Shoot, M, Braye, S, Preston, O, Allen, K and Spreadbury, K (2020) *Analysis of Safeguarding Adult Reviews April 2017–March 2019: Findings for Sector-led Improvement*. [online] Available at: https://tinyurl.com/2s3s4a2j (accessed 13 November 2024).

Procter, P M and Wilson, M L (2018) Nursing, Professional Curiosity and Big Data Cocreating eHealth in Building Continents of Knowledge. In A Ugon, D Karlsson, G O Klein and A Moen (eds), *Oceans of Data: The Future of Co-Created eHealth* (pp 186–90). Amsterdam: European Federation for Medical Informatics (EFMI) and IOS Press.

R [2011] EWHC 1704 (Fam).

Rawles, J (2023) Critical Thinking and Reflective Practice. In J Parker (ed), *Introducing Social Work*. London: Sage.

Re ZK (No 2) [2021] EWCOP 61, paragraph 19.

Reder, P, Duncan, S and Gray, M (1993) *Beyond Blame: Child Abuse Tragedies Revisited*. London: Brunner-Routledge.

Rees, K (2023) *James: A Safeguarding Adults Review Using Rapid Methodology*. Teeswide Safeguarding Adult Board. [online] Available at: https://tinyurl.com/59rzrcs2 (accessed 13 November 2024).

Revell, L and Burton, V (2016) Supervision and the Dynamics of Collusion: A Rule of Optimism? *The British Journal of Social Work*, 46(6): 1587–601.

Riess, H (2017) The Science of Empathy. *Journal of Patient Experience*, 4(2): 74–7. https://doi.org/10.1177/2374373517699267.

Robinson, O C (2023) Probing in Qualitative Research Interviews: Theory and Practice. *Qualitative Research in Psychology*, 20(3): 382–97. https://doi.org/10.1080/14780887.2023.2238625.

Robson, C (2024) *Safeguarding Adult Review – Gerry*. Cornwall and Isles of Scilly Adult Safeguarding Board. [online] Available at: https://tinyurl.com/2u5p4svj (accessed 13 November 2024).

Roman, B (2011) Curiosity: A Best Practice in Education. *Medical Education*, 45: 654–6. https://doi.org/10.1111/j.1365-2923.2011.04017.x.

Ruck Keene, A, Kane, N B, Kim, S Y H and Owen, G S (2019) Taking Capacity Seriously? Ten Years of Mental Capacity Disputes Before England's Court of Protection. *International Journal of Law and Psychiatry*, 62: 56–76. https://doi.org/10.1016/j.ijlp.2018.11.005.

Ryakhovskaya, Y, Jach, H K and Smillie, L D (2022) Curiosity as Feelings of Interest versus Deprivation: Relations Between Curiosity Traits and Affective States When Anticipating Information. *Journal of Research in Personality*, 96: 104164.

Sabanciogullari, S, Yilmaz, F T and Karabey, G (2021) The Effect of the Clinical Nurse's Compassion Levels on Tendency to Make Medical Errors: A Cross-sectional Study. *Contemporary Nurse*, 57: 65–79. https://doi.org/10.1080/10376178.2021.1927772.

Sahota, P (2023) *Adult K Safeguarding Adult Review Executive Summary*. Teeswide Safeguarding Adult Board (TSAB). [online] Available at: https://tinyurl.com/fuk9r88b (accessed 13 November 2024).

Sandiford, A (2023a) *Safeguarding Adult Review, Adult L*. Rochdale Borough Safeguarding Adults Boards. [online] Available at: https://tinyurl.com/3z7rr6sx (accessed 13 November 2024).

Sandiford, A (2023b) *Safeguarding Adult Review, Adult H*, Rochdale Borough Safeguarding Adults Boards. [online] Available at: https://tinyurl.com/3a2whx78 (accessed 13 November 2024).

Santos Meneses, L (2020) Critical Thinking Perspectives Across Contexts and Curricula: Dominant, Neglected, and Complementing Dimensions. *Thinking Skills and Creativity*, 35: 100610. https://doi.org/10.1016/j.tsc.2019.100610.

Scottish Government (2019) *Adult Support and Protection Improvement Plan 2019–22*. [online] Available at: https://tinyurl.com/y6y284ew (accessed 13 November 2024).

Senker, S, Eason, A, Pawson, C and McCartan, K (2023) *Issues, Challenges and Opportunities for Trauma-informed Practice*. HM Inspectorate of Probation. [online] Available at: https://tinyurl.com/3cjc9szh (accessed 13 November 2024).

Seth, A (2021) *Being You: A New Science of Consciousness*. London: Faber and Faber.

Seth, A (2024) *Consciousness in Humans and in Other Things*. [online] Available at: https://tinyurl.com/m6hmvm6m (accessed 13 November 2024).

Siegel, D J (2020) *The Developing Mind: How Relationships and the Brain Interact to Shape Who We Are*, 3rd ed. New York: Guilford Press.

Simmons, C (2019) *Safeguarding Adults Review in Respect of MS*. West Sussex Safeguarding Adults Board. [online] Available at: https://tinyurl.com/4r4z72u7 (accessed 13 November 2024).

Singer, T and Klimecki, O M (2014) Empathy and Compassion. *Current Biology*, 24(18): R875–78. https://doi.org/10.1016/j.cub.2014.06.054.

Skills for Care (2024) Turning Point for Social Care as the Sector Launches a Workforce Strategy. [online] Available at: https://tinyurl.com/ycyyjmdp (accessed 13 November 2024).

Smith, E and El-Kaddah, J (2020) Richmond and Wandsworth Safeguarding Adult Board Harvey. [online] Available at: https://tinyurl.com/yyd3wucw (accessed 13 November 2024).

Social Work England (2020) Professional Standards. [online] Available at: www.socialworkengland.org.uk/standards/professional-standards (accessed 14 August 2024).

Social Services and Wellbeing (Wales) Act 2014. [online] Available at: www.legislation.gov.uk/anaw/2014/4/contents (accessed 13 November 2024).

Solihull Safeguarding Adults Board (2018) *SAR Stephen* [online] Available at: www.safeguardingsolihull.org.uk/ssab/safeguarding-adult-reviews/safeguarding-adult-review-reports (accessed 13 November 2024).

Somani, S (2005) Cultural Curiosity. *PM Network Magazine*, 19(1): 66.

Spányik, A, Simon, D, Rigó, A, Griffiths, M D and Demetrovics, Z (2023) Emotional Exhaustion and Traumatic Stress Among Healthcare Workers During the COVID-19 Pandemic: Longitudinal Changes and Protective Factors. *PLoS One*, 18(12): e0291650. https://doi.org/10.1371/journal.pone.0291650.

Spreadbury, K (2021) *Rotherham Safeguarding Adults Board Safeguarding Adult Review The Painter and His Son*. [online] Available at: https://tinyurl.com/2dxjn2u5 (accessed 13 November 2024).

Spreadbury, K and Buckland, R (2021) *Safeguarding Adults Review: Learning from the Circumstances Around the Death of Five Women in Gloucestershire*. Gloucestershire Safeguarding Adults Boards. [online] Available at: https://tinyurl.com/2y4fud99 (accessed 13 November 2024).

Spreadbury, K and Hubbard, R (2020) *The Adult Safeguarding Practice Handbook*. Bristol: Policy Press.

Spreadbury, K and Lawson, J (2021) *Deciding If You Need to Raise a Safeguarding Concern to the Local Authority*: Multi-Agency Safeguarding Hub (MASH). Local Government Association (LGA) and the Association of Directors of Adult Social Services (ADASS). [online] Available at: www.local.gov.uk/sites/default/files/documents/25.168_Understanding_what_constitutes_a_safeguarding_07.1.pdf (accessed 13 November 2024).

Stanley, S and Webber, M (2022) Systematic Review of Service User and Carer Involvement in Qualifying Social Work Education: A Decade in Retrospect. *The British Journal of Social Work*, 52(8): 4871–93. https://doi.org/10.1093/bjsw/bcac080.

Starns, B (2019) *Safeguarding Adults Together Under the Care Act 2014: A Multi-agency Practice Guide*. St Albans: Critical Publishing.

Stevens, E, Price, L and Walker, L (2022) Just Because People are Old, Just Because They're Ill ... Dignity Matters in District Nursing. *Journal of Adult Protection*, 24, 3–14.

Strauss, C, Lever Taylor, B, Gu, J, Kuyken, W, Baer, R, Jones, F and Cavanagh, K (2016) What is Compassion and How Can We Measure It? A Review of Definitions and Measures. *Clinical Psychological Review*, 47: 15–27. https://doi.org/10.1016/j.cpr.2016.05.004.

Swindon Safeguarding Partnership (2023) *Safeguarding Adult Review Brenda*. [online] Available at: https://tinyurl.com/mr27fa9a (accessed 13 November 2024).

Tameside Adults Safeguarding Partnership Board (2023). *Safeguarding Adult Review: RE Gaynor*. [online] Available at: https://nationalnetwork.org.uk/2023/Gaynor-SAR.pdf (accessed 13 November 2024).

Tanner, D (2020) The Love That Dare Not Speak Its Name: The Role of Compassion in Social Work Practice. *The British Journal of Social Work*, 50(6): 1688–705. https://doi.org/10.1093/bjsw/bcz 127.

Thacker, H, Anka, A and Penhale, B (2020) *Professional Curiosity in Safeguarding Adults: Strategic Briefing*. Dartington: Research in Practice.

Thacker, H, Anka, A and Penhale, B (2019) Could Curiosity Save Lives? An Exploration into the Value of Employing Professional Curiosity and Partnership Work in Safeguarding Adults Under the *Care Act 2014*. *Journal of Adult Protection*, 21(5): 252–67. https://doi.org/10.1108/JAP-04-2019-0014.

The Safeguarding Vulnerable Groups (NI) Order (2007) [online] Available at: www.legislation.gov.uk/nisi/2007/1351/contents (accessed 13 November 2024).

Tinto, V. (2017) Reflections on Student Persistence. *Student Success,* 8(2): 1–6. https://doi.org/10.5204/ssj.v8i2.376.

Tuominen, J Tölli, S Häggman, L A (2023) Violence by Clients and Patients Against Social and Healthcare Staff: An Integrative Review of Staff's Well-being at Work, Implementation of Work and Leaders' Activities. *Journal of Clinical Nursing* 32(13): 3173–84. https://doi.org/10.1111/jocn.16425.

Turner, D and Fanner, M (2022) *Digital Connection in Health and Social Work: Perspectives from COVID-19*. St Albans: Critical Publishing.

Violence Against Women, Domestic Abuse and Sexual Violence (Wales) Act 2015. [online] Available at: www.legislation.gov.uk/anaw/2015/3/contents (accessed 13 November 2024).

Vogel, S and Flint, B (2021) Compassionate Leadership: How to Support Your Team When Fixing the Problem Seems Impossible. *Nursing Management,* 28(1): 32–41. https://doi.org/10.7748/nm.2021.e1967.

Wang, G, Albayrak, A, Hogervorst, E and van der Cammen, T J M (2021) Know-Me: A Toolkit for Designing Personalised Dementia Care. *International Journal of Environmental Research in Public Health,* 18(11): 5662. https://doi.org/10.3390/ijerph18115662.

Ward, M (2023) *Safeguarding Adult Review – Keith*. Manchester Safeguarding Partnership. [online] Available at: https://tinyurl.com/yu4s9m7a (accessed 13 November 2024).

Ward, M (2024) *Safeguarding Adult Review – Thomas*. Gateshead Safeguarding Adult Board. [online] Available at: https://tinyurl.com/3jkkmwzj (accessed 13 November 2024).

Waring, S and Jones, A (2023) Cost–benefit Analysis of Partnership Working Between Fire and Rescue and Health Services Across England and Wales During the COVID-19 Pandemic. *British Medical Journal,* 13(7): e072263. https://doi.org/10.1136/bmjopen-2023-072263.

Warrington Borough Council v Y & Ors [2023] EWCOP 27.

Weinstein, N, Itzchakov, G and Legate, N (2022) The Motivational Value of Listening During Intimate and Difficult Conversations. *Social and Personality Psychology Compass*, 16: e12651. https://doi.org/10.1111/spc3.12651.

Weisz, E and Cikara, M (2021) Strategic Regulation of Empathy. *Trends in Cognitive Sciences*, 25(3): 213–27. https://doi.org/10.1016/j.tics.2020.12.002.

West Berkshire Safeguarding Adults Board (2023) *Safeguarding Adults Review 7 Minute Learning Summary John*. [online] Available at: https://tinyurl.com/3nbmr5aw (accessed 13 November 2024).

Whitecross, W M and Smithson, M (2023) Curiously Different: Interest-curiosity and Deprivation-curiosity May Have Distinct Benefits and Drawbacks. *Personality and Individual Differences*, 213: 112310. https://doi.org/10.1016/j.paid.2023.112310.

Whitecross, W M and Smithson, M (2023a) Open or Opposed to Unknowns: How Do Curious People Think and Feel About Uncertainty? *Personality and Individual Differences,* 209: 112210. https://doi.org/10.1016/j.paid.2023.112210.

Whitehead, S (2023) *Discretionary Safeguarding Adults Review (Tina)*. West Berkshire Safeguarding Adults Board. [online] Available at: https://tinyurl.com/mt55asns (accessed 13 November 2024).

Whitlock, J and Purington, M (2013) *Respectful Curiosity*. Ithaca, NY: Cornell University Press.

Wilkins, D (2024) Seven Principles of Effective Supervision for Child and Family Social Work. *Practice*, 36(3): 213–29. https://doi.org/10.1080/09503153.2023.2261148.

Williams, S and Bateman, F (2022) *Safeguarding Adult Review, Philip*. City and Hackney Safeguarding Adults Board. [online] Available at: https://tinyurl.com/mt46vwd7 (accessed 13 November 2024).

Williams, D P and Chisholm, T (2018) Reflections on a Serious Case Review: How Health Recommendations Have Changed Since 2011 and the Impact of Professional Curiosity on Health Assessments. *Adoption & Fostering*, 42(2): 201–5.

Winter, M (2021) *Safeguarding Adults Review Learning from the Circumstances of the death of 'Peter'*. Gloucestershire Safeguarding Adults Board. [online] Available at: https://nationalnetwork.org.uk/2021/Peter.pdf (accessed 13 November 2024).

Wirral Safeguarding Children Partnership (2022) *Child Safeguarding Practice Review, Child Q*. [online] Available at: https://tinyurl.com/436ybn3e (accessed 13 November 2024).

World Health Organisation (WHO, 2021) *COVID-19 and the Social Determinants of Health and Health Equity: Evidence Brief*. Geneva: WHO.

Yager, J and Kay, J (2020) Clinical Curiosity in Psychiatric Residency Training: Implications for Education and Practice. *Academic Psychiatry,* 44: 90–94. https://doi.org/10.1007/s40596-019-01131-w.

Yan, E, Lai, D W L, Sun, R, Cheng, S T, Ng, H K L, Lou, V W Q and Kwok, T (2023) Typology of Family Caregivers of Older Persons: A Latent Profile Analysis Using Elder Mistreatment Risk and Protective Factors. *Journal of Elder Abuse & Neglect,* 35(1): 34–64. https://doi.org/10.1080/08946566.2023.2197269.

Yardley, E (2020) Technology-facilitated Domestic Abuse in Political Economy: A New Theoretical Framework. *Violence Against Women,* 27(10): 107780122094717. https://doi.org/10.1177/1077801220947172.

Ylönen, K (2023) The Use of Electronic Information Systems in Social Work: A Scoping Review of the Empirical Articles Published Between 2000 and 2019. *European Journal of Social Work,* 26(3): 575–88. https://doi.org/10.1080/13691457.2022.2064433.

Young, L (2023) *Child X Local Child Safeguarding Practice Review.* Gloucestershire Safeguarding Children's Partnership (GSCP). [online] Available at: https://tinyurl.com/be37c7j3 (accessed 13 November 2024).

Zedelius, C M, Gross, M E and Schooler, J W (2022) Inquisitive but Not Discerning: Deprivation Curiosity is Associated with Excessive Openness to Inaccurate Information. *Journal of Research in Personality,* 98: 104227.

Zhu, C, Kwok, N T K, Chan, T C W, Chan, G H K and So, S H W (2021) Inflexibility in Reasoning: Comparisons of Cognitive Flexibility, Explanatory Flexibility, and Belief Flexibility Between Schizophrenia and Major Depressive Disorder. *Frontiers in Psychiatry,* 11: 609569.

Index

Page numbers in *italics* refer to figures. Page numbers in **bold** refer to tables.

active listening, 68, 105
Adult Support and Protection (Scotland) Act (2007), 101
adultification bias, 32, 81
adverse childhood experiences, 70
advocacy, 92, 94–5, 97, 99, 106
affective empathy, 106
algorithmic decision-making, 118
Allen, M, 48
ambiguity, 6, 11, 15
anchoring bias, 32
Anstiss, T, 110
Anthony, W, 123
Appleton, J V, 20, 39, 107
artificial intelligence (AI), 118
assumptions, 25, 31–3, 37, 42, 51, 72, 73, 80–1, 108, 124
austerity, 40
autonomy, 41, 79, 96
Aven, T, 128
avoiders, **9**

Baillie L, 134
Bansal, A, 11, 12
Barnett, D, 17
Barnsley Safeguarding Adults Board, 136
Barrett, L F, 48, 50
barriers to professional curiosity, **25–6** 20–1, 23, 24, 25–8
   case dynamics, 34–6
   organisational issues, 36–40
   personal issues, 28–34
   systemic factors, 40–2
Bateman, F, 40
Behan-Devlin, J, 118, 119
Bernard, 111
best practices, 123
   personalised trauma-informed approaches, 132–4
   rapport-building and persistence, 135–7
   risk assessment, 123–30
   trauma-informed approaches, 131–4
Bexley, 76
bias
   cognitive, 31–2, 45, 56, 58

confirmation, 47, 50, 56, 57
   in multi-agency setting, 77
   personal, 31–3, 80–1, 124
   unconscious, 46
bodily sensations, 48, 50, *51*, 51–2, 55
body scan, 55, 61
Boryczko, M, 108
Botham, 112
brain, 45–6, 47–8, 50, 56
Braye, S, 15
Britten, S, 35, 62, 124
Broadhurst, K, 62
Brookfield, K, 134
Buckland, R, 132
bureaucratic processes, 36
Burnard, P, 105
burnout, 26, 28–9, 38
Burton, V, 11, 28, 29, 37, 42, 80

Calvard, T, 106
capacity assessment. *See under* mental capacity
Care Act (2014), 88, 91, 137
   and Safeguarding Adults Boards, 88–9
   section 42, safeguarding adult duties under, **89**, 89–90
   Statutory Guidance Accompanying the Care Act 2014, 93
   well-being checklist, 89–90
Care and Support Statutory Guidance, 91, 124
carer's assessment, 90
Carr, S, 25
case coordination, 115
case dynamics, **26**
   disguised compliance, 35
   knowing but not knowing, 36
   limited knowledge base, 34–5
   normalisation, 36
   rule of optimism, 35
case history, 55–6, 57, 60, 63, 80, 118
caseloads, 28–9, 37–9
Chatfield, T, 56
Chisholm, T, 11, 17, 20
Cikara, M, 106
City and Hackney Safeguarding Adults Board, 38

clarification probes, 112
Clark, A, 46, 48
clearinghouse probes, 112
Climbie, V, 10
Climbie, Victoria, 15, 36
Cocker, 29
cognitive bias, 31–2, 45, 56, 58
cognitive overload, 50
communication, 66, 77, 92, 105, 127
    and digital technology, 117
    probes/probing, 110–13
    skills, 11, 39, 72
compassion, 55, 105, 109–10, 115, 137, 139
compassion fatigue, 29
Compassion in the Workplace model, 110
confidence, lack of, 33–4
    fear of making mistakes, 33–4
    fear of reaction, 33–4
    professional deference, 34
confirmation bias, 31, 47, 50, 56, 57
consensus probes, 112
content-oriented listeners, **67**
contextual external probes, 111
continuing professional development, 39, 59
Court of Protection (COP), 95, 97, 117
covert social curiosity, **8**
Covid-19 pandemic, 2, 28, 114, 117
Cramphorn, K, 20
Criminal Law Act (NI) (1967), 101
critical analysis, 49, 59, 62, 105, 108–9
critical mindset, 55, 56
critical reflection, 49, 105
critical thinking, 6, 105, 108–9
cultural curiosity, 33, 105, 124
curiosity, 6–7, 9, 11, 136, 138
    cultural, 33, 105, 124
    as deprivation, 7
    empathic, 17
    epistemic, 6
    as a feeling of interest, 7
    five dimensions of, **7–8**
    importance in safeguarding work, 10
    types of curious people, **8–9**, 8

data-generation activities in organisations, 21
Data Protection Act (2018), 100
Davidson, G, 102
Davis, J, 32, 81
decisional capacity assessment, 96–9
decision-making, 31, 45, 55, 90, 105, 124, 137
    and compassion fatigue, 29
    and curiosity, 10
    and emotions, 48, 61
    and mental capacity, 94–100
    and professional curiosity, 17
    multidisciplinary, 81
    shared, 90, 128
Delgado N, 106

Depow, G, 106
Deprivation of Liberty Safeguards (DoLs), 94, 100
Deprivation Sensitivity (curiosity dimension), **8**
deprivation-type curiosity, 7
Devlin, 118
DICE approach to probing, 111
Dickens, J, 24, 39, 41, 59
difficult conversations, holding, 54–5, 61, 82
digital technology, 2, 117–20, 134
disguised compliance, 13, 35, 55
dispositional interest-curiosity, 7
domestic abuse, 61, 134
Domestic Abuse Act (2021), 100
Domestic Abuse and Civil Proceedings Act (Northern Ireland) (2021), 101
Domestic Abuse, Stalking, Harassment and Honour Based Violence Assessment (DASH), 134

economically driven partnership work, 85
Efilti, P, 106
Egan, 111
electronic health information exchange platform, 134
electronic information systems (EIS), 117, 118, 119
emotional exhaustion, 26, 28–9
emotions, 7, 48, 50, 61, 106, 109, 110, 112
empathic curiosity, 17
empathisers, **9**
empathy, 11, 12, 55, 69, 72, 92, 105–7, 137
enablers of professional curiosity, 93
    case example, 60–2
    characteristics/attributes that foster curiosity practice, 45
    curious organisational culture, 58–9
    holding difficult conversations, 54–5, 61
    impact of prior experiences, 46–7, 48–50
    information gathering, 55–8, 60
    practices that support curiosity, 50–3
    predictive processing, 45–6, 48
    reflective questions to support practitioners, 62–3
    role of emotions, 48
    role of managers, 59–60
    self-care, 53–4
enduring power of attorney, 94
England, 14, 17, 88, 94, **102**, 114, 117
epistemic curiosity, 6
Equality Act (2010), 100, 101, 132
evidence, 1, 17, 18, 35, 56, 57, 58, 61, 62, 76
    -based practice, 17, 47, 123, 130
    visual, 73
executive functioning, 73, 75, 96–9
exemplification probes, 112
explanatory probes, 111–12
extension probes, 111
external descriptive probes, 111

family, 24, 75, 112
    abuse in intra-familial relationships, 92
    dynamics, 12–13, 138

'think family' approach, 114
unpaid carers, safeguarding of, 15
Farkas, M, 123
fascinators, **8**, 135
Feldon, P, 100
felt sense, 47, 48, 50, 51–2
Ferguson, H, 36
fight or flight response, 50
Flint, B, 110, 113, 115
Frame, H, 80
Fynn, J F, 85

Gelmez, K, 106
Gilbert, P, 109
Gorden, 111
grounding skills, 131
groupthink, 58
growth mindset, 11
gut feelings, 52, 55, 62, 76

Hafford-Letchfield, T, 25, 92
Hargie, 67
Health and Care Act (2022), 100
healthy scepticism, 15, 55
Hilgartner, S, 123
honesty, 30, 55, 69, 82
Hopkinson, P, 86
hot cross bun reflective tool, *51*, 51–2
Human Rights Act (1989), 100
Human Rights Act (1998), 17, 97, 101, 137
Hutson, M, 48

Independent Mental Capacity Advocate (IMCA), 94–5, 97, 99
indeterminacy, 15
information, 17
gap, 6, 7, 39, 111
gathering, 18, 55–8, 60, 89, 133
'Know me' digital toolkit, 134
personal information documents, 133–4
sharing, 70, 115, 117, 119, 133, 134
information technology (IT) systems, 80
integrative thinking, 128
inter-agency collaboration, 114–17, 133
interest-type curiosity, 7
internal description probes, 112
intra-familial relationships, and abuse, 92
intuition, 1, 124

Jeyasingham, 118
joint visits, 60, 133
Joss, 29
joyous exploration (curiosity dimension), **7**

Kahneman, D, 51
Kashdan, T B, 6, **8**, 8–9, 10, 45
Kay, J, 6
key worker, 133

King Jr, S H, 106
Klimecki, O M, 109
'Know me' digital toolkit, 134
knowledge
base, limited, 34–5
epistemic curiosity, 6
gap, 111
Korteling, J E, 56
Ku, G, 106

Lacy, R, 58
Laming, W H, 10, 11, 15
language, 48, 81
lasting powers of attorney, 94
Lawson, J, 90
leadership, 59, 60, 116, 137
learning, 59–60
continuing learning development, 115
and curiosity, 6, 134
learning partnership work model, 85
Leeds Safeguarding Adults Board, 110
legal framework for safeguarding adults, 87, 100, 102
Care Act (2014), 88–90
in England, 88
in Scotland, 101
international comparisons, 102
Mental Capacity (Amendment) Act (2019), 99–100
Mental Capacity Act (2005), 94–5, **95**
Mental Health Act (1983), 93–4
in Northern Ireland, 101
Safeguarding Adults Boards, 88–9
in Wales, 100–1
Leigh, J, 35
Liberty Protection Safeguards (LPS), 99, 100
listening, 1, 6, 12, 13, 17, 68–70, 92, 105, 106, 107
active, 68, 105
high-quality, 68
types of listeners, **67**
Litman, J A, 7
Loewenstein, G, 6

Making Safeguarding Personal (MSP), 14, 90, 91–3, 115, 123
managers, 59–60, 62, 63, 115, 137
Manchester Safeguarding Partnership, 115
Marsh, N, 32, 81
Martin, R, 128
Maynard, E, 20
media, 40, 42
meetings
multi-agency, 77, 115
virtual, 2, 21, 118
mental capacity, 72–3, 74, 78, 94–5, **95**, 99–100, 102, 107
assessment, 95–100
presumption of capacity, 95, 98

Mental Capacity (Amendment) Act (2019), 99–100
Mental Capacity Act (MCA, 2005), 94–5, **95**, 96, **96–7**, 97, 98, 99
Mental Health Act (1983), 94
mental models, 45
mindfulness practice, 53, 55
mobile devices, 117, 119
Mooney images, 47–8
Muirden, C E, 20, 39, 107
Multi Agency Risk Assessment Conference (MARAC), 134
multi-agency management groups, 116
Multi-Agency Safeguarding Trackers (MAST), 117
multi-agency setting, professional curiosity in, 67, 75–9
   examples of, 77–9
   professional difficulties and escalating concerns, 77

need assessment, 90
negotiation skills, 105
New Zealand, 102
Nicolas, J, 54
Norfolk Safeguarding Adults Board, 30, 36
normalisation, 36, 47, 74
Northern Ireland, 100, 101, **102**
nudging probes, 111

Open Justice Court of Protection, 2
open questions, 11, 72, 82
organisational issues, **26**
   bureaucratic processes, 36
   inadequate supervision, 37
   insufficient training and development, 39–40
   resource constraints, 37–8
   time pressure, 37, 38–9
   workload pressure, 37–9
organisations, 28, 63, 137
   and professional curiosity, 20–1, 59–60
   organisational culture, 39, 42, 58–9
   and staff abuse, 30
Osburn, O, 123
overt social curiosity, **8**
oxygen mask theory, 30

Parker, J, 123
partnership work, 61, 66, 76, 84–5, 123
   and digital technology, 117–20
   capacity assessment, 95–9
   compassion, 109–10
   core skills underpinning, 105
   critical thinking and analysis, 108–9
   effective, characteristics of, **87**
   empathy, 105–7
   importance in safeguarding work, 85–6
   inter-agency collaboration, 114–17, 133
   involvement of other professionals, 113–14
   involvement of PWLE, 107
   legal framework for safeguarding adults, 87–90, 100–1, 102

Making Safeguarding Personal (MSP) initiative, 91–3
   and Mental Capacity Act (2005), 94–5, **95**
   and Mental Capacity (Amendment) Act (2019), 99–100
   and Mental Health Act (1983), 94
   models, 85
   probes/probing, 110–13
Patel, 38
peer debriefing, 31
people with lived experiences (PWLE), 12
   involvement in safeguarding work, 14, 107, 137
   and professional curiosity, 12–14, 138
people-oriented listeners, **67**
Percy-Smith, J, 85
perseverance, 135
persistence, 135–7
Personal and Property Rights Act 1998 (PPPR Act), New Zealand, 102
personal history, 17, 133
personal information documents, 133–4
personal issues, **25**, 28
   compassion fatigue, 29
   emotional exhaustion and burnout, 28–9
   lack of confidence, 33–4
   personal bias and assumptions, 31–3, 80–1
   secondary trauma, 29–31
personalised trauma-informed approaches, 132–4
person-centred approach, 25, 90, 91, 128, 132
person-centred partnership work, 85
perspective-taking, 1, 105, 106–7
Phillips, J, 11, 25, 28, 40, 82
power relations, 33, 75, 81
practice tips, 79–82
prediction errors, 45, 46, 48, 50, 51, 56
predictive processing, 45–6, 48
Preston-Shoot, M, 24, 36, 124, 128, 138
presumption of capacity, 95, 98
principles underpinning safeguarding adults, **91**, 93, 124
prior experiences, 50, 51, 53, 54, 56, 70
   and emotions, 48
   impact on predictions, 46–7, 48–50
probes/probing, 12, 110–13
   questions, 33, 66, 72
   taxonomy of, 111
problem-solvers, **9**
proceduralisation, 39, 42
Procter, P M, 17, 21
professional dangerousness, 13, 138
professional deference, 34
Professional, Statutory and Regulatory Bodies (PSRBs), 2
prompt questions, 96
Purington, M, 12

questions, 1, 12, 13, 15, 17, 24, 33, 35, 127, 139

open, 11, 72, 82
probing, 12, 33, 66, 72
prompt, 96
self-reflective, 35
to support practitioners, 62–3

rapport-building, 24, 68, 76, 95, 135–7
Rawles, J, 108
reasonable adjustments, 132
Reder, 28
Rees, K, 132, 133 33–4
referrals, 116, 133
reflective practice, 30, 37, 62, 72
relationship-building, 1, 15, 24, 37, 41, 60, 66, 68, 70, 76, 95, 107, 110, 124
remote work, 2, 118
resource constraints in organisations, 37–8, 40
respectful curiosity, 11–12
respectful uncertainty, 15
retraumatisation, 131, 133
Revell, L, 11, 28, 29, 37, 42, 80
Riess, H, 106
right to life, 17
risk assessment, 55, 77, 118, 123, 134, 136
    inter-agency, 134
    limitations of risk assessment and impact matrix, 127
    risk analysis, 127–8
    risk assessment and impact matrix, 124, **125–6**
    risk evaluation, 129–30
    risk-identification assessment, 107, 124–7
    stages of, **130–1**
risk-enablement plans, 107, 111, 117, 134
risk management, 45, 77, 115, 117, 130, 134
Robinson, O C, 111
Robson, C, 109
Roman, B, 6
routine enquiry, 61
Ruck Keene, A, 97
rule of optimism, 35, 37

safe space, 37, 99, 131
safe uncertainty, 15
Safeguarding Adults Boards (SABs), 66, 77, 88–9
Safeguarding Adults Collection (SAC), 92
safeguarding apps, 119
Safeguarding Vulnerable Groups (NI) Order (2007), 101
safety plans, 92
Santos Meneses, L, 108
scamming, and digital technology, 119
Scotland, 100, 101, **102**
secondary trauma, 29–31, 70
self-awareness, 11, 46, 49, 50–1, 110, 124
self-care, 17, 53–4
self-neglect, 31, 36, 60, 68, 73, 74, 86
self-reports, 24, 69, 119
Seth, A, 48
shame, 15, 105

sine wave speech, 47, 48
Singer, T, 109
Singh, 38
skills, in professional curiosity, 18, **19–20**, 105
social curiosity, **8**, 15
Social Services and Wellbeing (Wales) Act (2014), 100–1
societal attitudes, 41–2
Spreadbury, K, 90, 132
staff
    abuse, 30
    turnover, 37, 38
    violence against, 33
Starns, B, 17, 18, 100
stereotyping, 31, 33, 81
Stevens, E, 138
stigma, 15, 41–2
Strauss C, 109
strengths-based approach, 60, 70, 90, 91, 93
stress
    and compassion fatigue, 29
    impact of, 50
    tolerance, **8**
supervision, 30, 37, 59, 63, 66, 76, 108, 124
surface acting, 28
Swindon Safeguarding Partnership Board, 85
systemic issues, **26**
    austerity, 40
    increasing demand for services, 41
    policy and legislative constraints, 41
    political and cultural context, 42
    societal attitudes and stigma, 41–2

Tanner, D, 109, 110
task-oriented listeners, **67**
team debriefing, 31
Teeswide Safeguarding Adults Board, 73, 132
text-based communication, 117
Thacker, H, 11, 20, 25, 36, 37, 59, 60, 118
therapeutic relationship, 11
'think family' approach, 114
'This is Me' (personal information document), 134
Thomas, N, 134
thrill seeking (curiosity dimension), **8**
time pressure, 37, 38–9, 67
time specific probes, 111
time-oriented listeners, **67**
Tinto, V, 135
Toet, A, 56
Tower Hamlets Safeguarding Adults Board, 123
training, 37, 39–40, 59–60, 61, 66, 107, 117, 137, 139
trauma, 75
    -informed approaches, 70–2, 128, 131–4
    secondary, 29–31, 70
trust, 1, 15, 41, 60, 68, 70, 95, 99, 105, 107, 110, 124, 132, 138

Tsakiris, T, 48
two-stage functional test, 96, **96–7**, 98, 100

uncertainty, 6, 11, 15, 76
   respectful, 15
   safe, 15
unconscious bias, 31–3, 46
unwise choices, 72–5

value-based practice, 123, 130
video conferencing, 117
Violence Against Women, Domestic Abuse and Sexual Violence (Wales) Act 2015, 100–1
virtual meetings, 2, 21, 118
Vogel S, 110, 113, 115

Wales, 94, 100–1, **102**, 114
Wales Safeguarding Procedures (2021), 101
Ward, M, 98, 115, 116
Warrington Borough Council v Y & Ors (2023), 95, 96
Weinstein, 68

Weisz, E, 106
West Sussex Safeguarding Adults Board, 110
WhatsApp, 117
Whitby, K, 35, 62, 124
Whitlock, J, 12
Wilkson, 37
Williams, D P, 11, 17, 20
Wilson, M L, 17, 21
window of tolerance, 131–2
work environment, 30, 58, 80
workload
   management, 41
   pressure, 28, 37–9, 40, 67

Yager, J, 6
Yan, E, 92
Yardley, E, 134
Ylönen, 118

Zedelius, C M, 7
zero tolerance approach to staff abuse, 30

Printed in the United States
by Baker & Taylor Publisher Services